AF598065

Training in Minimal Access Surgery

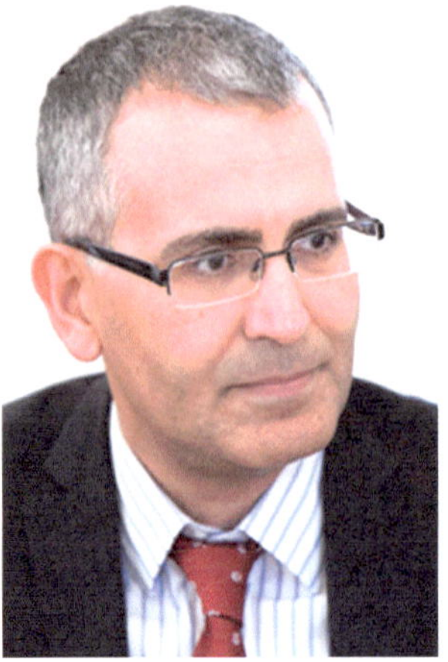

Nader Francis

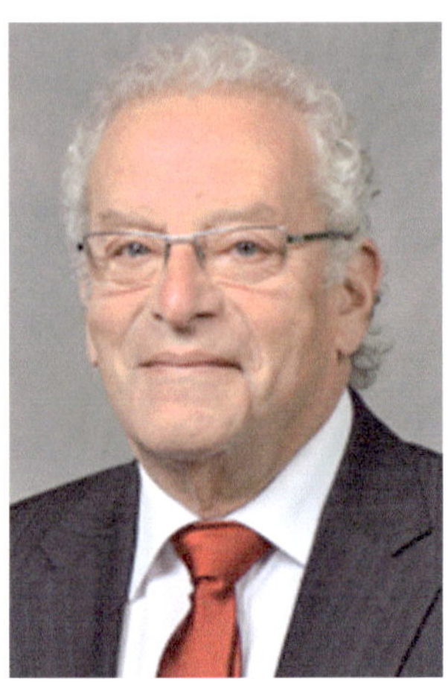

Abe Fingerhut

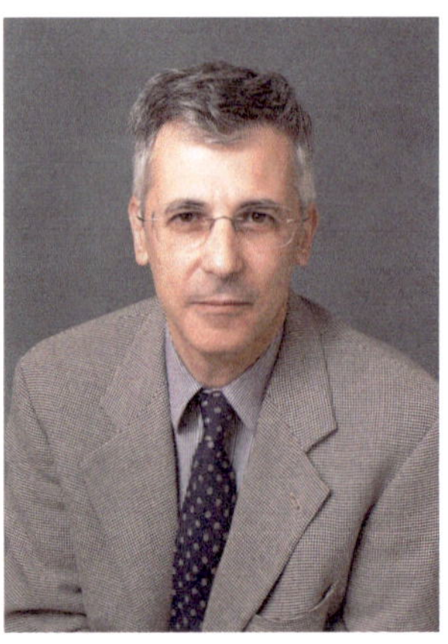

Roberto Bergamaschi

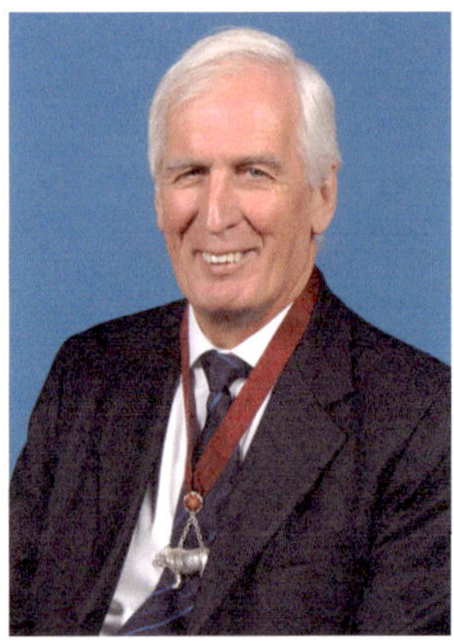

Roger Motson

Nader Francis • Abe Fingerhut
Roberto Bergamaschi • Roger Motson
Editors

Training in Minimal Access Surgery

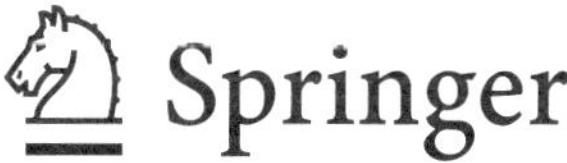

Editors
Nader Francis
NHS Foundation Trust
Yeovil District Hospital
Yeovil
UK

Abe Fingerhut
Poissy Cedex
France

Roberto Bergamaschi
Stony Brook Medicine
New York, NY
USA

Roger Motson
Colchester General Hospital
Colchester, Essex
UK

ISBN 978-1-4471-6493-7 ISBN 978-1-4471-6494-4 (eBook)
DOI 10.1007/978-1-4471-6494-4

Library of Congress Control Number: 2015948218

Springer London Heidelberg New York Dordrecht

Printed on acid-free paper

Springer-Verlag London Ltd. is part of Springer Science+Business Media (www.springer.com)

Preface

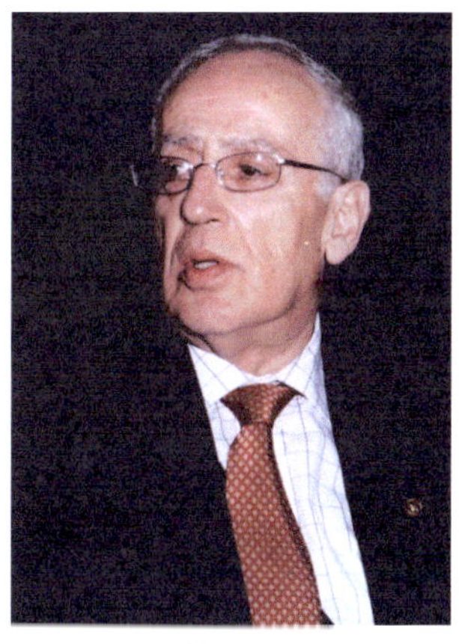

I readily accepted the task to write this Preface for several reasons, but primarily because it addresses a topic of seminal importance to the surgical profession. This book stresses concepts which I have always considered as conceptually valid and important throughout my career, such as *minimal access surgery* (MAS), that is 'surgery designed to reduce the trauma of access', rather that the *semantically* incorrect *minimally invasive surgery*. Likewise the use of *learning curve* is not appropriate to describe the complex process by which a trainee surgeon reaches the quasi-automatic stress-free stage, when he or she is able to perform a specific operation consistently well with good patient outcome. The *proficiency-gain curve* goes well beyond 'learning' and is at the heart of modern competence-based training and underpins the importance of this book.

There is no doubt that the 13 chapters of *Training in Minimal Access Surgery* provide an excellent account of the advances that have been made in the subject since the advent of MAS in the mid-1980s; in this respect, this book contains a wealth of up-to-date information. Obviously, one expects to encounter some repetition with the involvement of so many authors, but I regard this in a positive light as reinforcement. Important issues such as Training Curriculum in MAS, Simulation and Training in MAS, Training for Trainers in Endoscopy (Colonoscopy), and several others are addressed in a scholarly, objective and detailed manner. I found the chapter on Teletraining in MAS to be particularly stimulating as it heralds the inexorable trend towards globalisation of training, inevitable in the digital age.

I complement the editors Dr. Francis, Dr. Fingerhut, Dr. Bergamaschi and Dr. Motson, all highly respected colleagues and indeed, all the authors for producing a much-needed account on training for MAS. I am sure it will be well received by the colleges and programme directors worldwide.

Prof Sir Alfred Cuschieri, FRSE
Chief Scientific Advisor, Institute for Medical Science
and Technology, University of Dundee

Contents

Chapter 1
Learning Environment and Setting Up a Training Unit in Minimal Access Surgery

Fiona Carter and Nader Francis

Introduction

Advanced Minimal Access Surgery (MAS) is technically challenging and within the context of its practice and training, the environment is often defiant. It can be marked by stress, responsibility and pressure that can negatively influence training and learning. As any surgery, MAS may sometimes be performed under suboptimal psychomotor conditions of sleep deprivation or following earlier, tiring operations. Additional pressures proper to MAS include financial targets and waiting lists. Yet public and professional expectations require that a surgeon is able to train junior colleagues, regardless of these difficulties. Managing the training environment requires the control of multiple inputs and demands during emergent situations. This chapter addresses all the attributes of the MAS training environment, how they could be optimised and how to set-up a training unit for MAS.

Optimum Training Environment

A training environment can be defined as the external condition(s) that can provide acquisition of knowledge, skills and competencies as a result of teaching in this field without compromising patient care. An optimum training environment is the one that promotes learning; supporting the improvement of performance and increasing the

F. Carter, BSc (Hons), PhD (✉)
Director of South West Surgical Training Network c.i.c., Yeovil, Somerset BA20 2RH, UK
e-mail: fjcarter@swstnic.org

N. Francis, MB ChB, PLAB, FRCS, PhD
Colorectal Surgery, Yeovil District Hospital NHS Foundation Trust,
Yeovil, Somerset BA21 4AT, UK
e-mail: Nader.francis@ydh.nhs.uk

N. Francis et al. (eds.), *Training in Minimal Access Surgery*,
DOI 10.1007/978-1-4471-6494-4_1

efficiency of the whole training process. This depends on whether the training is aimed for cognitive, technical (in or outside Operating Room (OR)) or behavioural coaching.

Before discussing the attributes of the optimum training environment, it is essential to first clarify the need for such a training environment in a complex and technically challenging intervention such as MAS. The simple answer is that a good training environment is likely to improve patient care. An optimum training environment is the setting that encourages optimum communication and team working between all the members of the OR team in order to facilitate learning, which promotes patient safety. A good educational case would also involve deconstructing the operation into tasks and subtasks where the teacher and the learner are aiming to optimamly performr each step of the operation- definitely this can only improve patients' outcome. An optimum training environment is therefore encouraged to promote safe operative performance, which ultimately improves patient care.

Examining the attributes of training environment has been traditionally focused on the technical skills in the OR, but more recently, attention has been paid on coaching human factors, cognitive and technical skills outside the OR.

For the purpose of discussion here, the training environment will be considered under physical environment and the educational environment in and outside OR.

Training Environment in the OR/Endoscopic Suite

Physical Environment

MAS is technology dependent and its wide adoption across many fields has been matched, and perhaps driven, by the rapid evolution of technology in this field.

Over the past few decades, MAS increasingly occurs in operating rooms equipped with advanced audio-visual technology, or what is referred to as "integrated operating rooms" (IOR), which include high-resolution video displays, touch-screen control, and digital information archiving, integrated into a purpose-built system that reduces dependence on mobile equipment. It is intended to increase efficiency in the OR and improve the ergonomics, communication and information systems for medical teams in any OR or endoscopy suite (Fig. 1.1).

Beyond facilitating the surgical procedure and improving efficiency, the integrated operating room facilitates live feeds to conference rooms and auditoriums for training and grand rounds. In addition, the integrated ORs have the potential to connect the surgeon for teaching and tele-monitoring at remote locations. The latter is discussed separately in Chap. 11, but briefly it involves remote coaching, whereby both the trainer and trainee are accessing live digital images of the operation, and the trainer can remotely coach surgeons through challenging parts of the surgery. However, technology needs to be matched at both sites to access the same quality of image with network cover of sufficient bandwidth to allow optimum audio and visual communication.

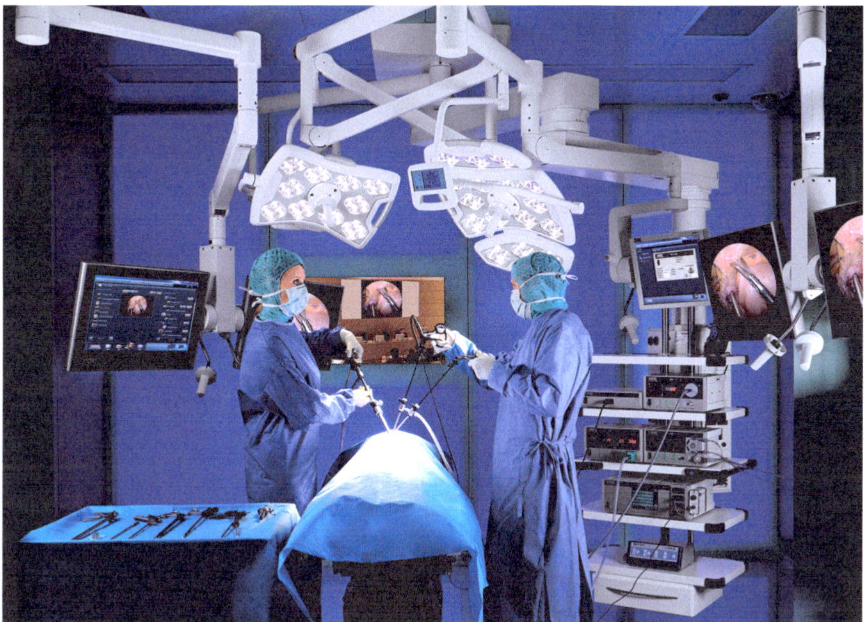

Fig. 1.1 Integrated OR (© KARL STORZ – Endoskope, Germany)

Training Environment

The primary focus of the OR team should always be patient safety and the effective performance of each procedure and these should also be the main objectives of both the trainer and trainee for a training case. However, training in the operating room should be conducted in an environment that is supportive to training and promote learning. Nevertheless, even with close supervision, inexperienced trainees will often take longer to perform a MAS procedure. This can create a conflict between the trainer, the trainee and the rest of the OR team. Dedicated operating training lists provide the best training environment in technically challenging surgery such as MAS. However, this warrants consideration of the financial pressures facing hospitals, with targets and the reduction of the training time (due to the adoption of European working time directive). Hence, these expectations and conflicts need to be addressed before, during and after the normal operating lists.

Before an operating list, the trainer needs to ensure the list is appropriately scheduled for training purposes and that the OR team are aware that some parts or the entire list will be used for training. Opportunity now exists, with the widespread use the WHO checklists, to address these issues and come to a common agreement and understanding for the whole team. During an operating list, the expectations and priorities of the trainee will need re-adjustment by the trainer if a case or cases have taken longer than expected. After completion of the case/ list, a

Table 1.1 Attributes of ideal training environment in the OR

1. Trainee-focused environment that supports learning
2. Unthreatening environment that allows the trainee and staff to ask questions and express opinion
3. Dedicated training list that allows time for training
4. Experienced professional staff who support training
5. Optimum selection of cases that suit the trainee's level
6. Supportive trainer who is a role model
7. Committed trainee who can make progress
8. Calm, quiet environment in theatre with minimal interruptions (phones, conversations, music etc.)
9. OR equipped with technology that facilitates feedback; such as video recording and image capture
10. Setting that allows confidential feedback after the training session when required

sign out process can allow the team to draw together the useful learning points that make future training cases run smoothly.

Attributes of an ideal training environment are summarised in Table 1.1. These may vary from the trainer, trainee and OR staff's point of view. The team brief is an ideal opportunity to discuss how the operating list should run for the mutual benefit of all and align all views of the entire team, in order to generate a safe environment for performance and training. Novices to MAS will be more susceptible to reduced performance in the presence of interference and the OR training environment should allow a trainee to focus on the task in hand with minimal interruptions.

Training Environment Outside the OR

A training environment outside the OR is designed to attain the attributes of ensuring a safe practice and optimum environment prior to undertaking surgery, usually through simulation techniques. One of the factors that underpin the success of a simulated training environment is the degree of realism where coaching is conducted. Technology is continually striving to provide an ever more realistic simulated environment for clinical training, which is resulting in very impressive systems. However, these systems are only available to a limited number of centres and thus to a limited number of learners. It will be necessary to be pragmatic about what facilities can be made available to the large numbers of surgical trainees who need to acquire MAS skills in a safe and effective manner. Very high fidelity learning environments will certainly have their place for the most advanced learners, multi-professional groups and perhaps for assessment and re-validation in the longer term. However, for the majority of learning episodes, it is unlikely to be possible to provide the highest level of realism.

When considering MAS, one could question the need for some elements that are included in a high fidelity simulated OR. For example, the room lights are often only used during the initial access and final closing aspect of a case. However, essential elements include:

1. Imaging equipment – actual laparoscope or static camera depends on the nature of the task. The more complex the task, the more advanced equipment are required for simulated training.
2. Surgical instruments – depends on the task; the whole range of instruments are required for instance to teach an advanced laparoscopic procedure, while a limited number is required to teach certain tasks such as laparoscopic suturing.
3. Simulations: this can involve a box trainer, virtual reality (VR) simulator synthetic or real animal parts, or human cadaver.

Training Environment in the Dry Lab

An ideal training environment for dry lab training should have enough space to allow free movement of tutors and delegates, with sufficient lighting and equipment. One could also argue that the space should be designed with a flexible set up that supports seminars, hands-on skills with audio-visual facilities and video links to the OR.

The requirements for the laparoscopic work-stations depend on the nature of the tasks; full laparoscopic stacks are required for advanced MAS but a minimum of a camera, light source, scope and training box are sufficient for more basic tasks. The simulated tasks can vary from a box with synthetic organs to ex-vivo animal tissue or hybrid simulations. There is wide use of VR simulators in the training of basic laparoscopic tasks of core procedures, but VR simulators with good validity for advanced laparoscopic surgery do not currently exist [1]. VR simulation still requires trainers to coach trainees on the simulated procedures and give constructive feedback [2].

Synthetic Simulations

There is a growing number of synthetic preparations, which often have a realistic anatomical appearances. The benefits of using these models include reproducibility, less requirement for specialist technical support and preparation, simple to store, low odour and are easy to dispose of. However, dissection of synthetic tissue is not as realistic and the material is either much stiffer or softer than that corresponding to the real task. Few of these models support the use of energised tissue dissection.

Ex-vivo Models

A compromise between synthetic models and live animal tissue is to create a hybrid of excised animal tissue mounted in specially designed frames. The aim is to fix the tissues in a position as close as possible to human anatomy [3–5]. The benefits are to improve the degree of realism and allow the use of tissue energisers. If ex-vivo animal organs are used, the environment should be designed such that surfaces are washable; adequate space and facilities to store and prepare and dispose of the materials is also necessary.

Wet Lab and Live Animal Lab

In the USA and some European countries, training using live animals is permitted. Whilst this approach provides realistic control of bleeding and tissue elasticity, there are many disadvantages: it is relatively expensive, due to the specialist facilities, staff and anaesthesia, and animal anatomy often differs significantly from humans, so the types of procedures that can be taught are limited. In addition to the growing ethical concerns, the use live animals for training is prohibited in the UK.

Cadaveric Training: Fresh Frozen and Thiel Embalmed

Despite the demonstrable benefits of integrating cadaver dissection into a resident training program [6, 7], cadaver surgery is not yet utilised in most training programmes due to the financial constraints and limitation of supply [8]. Cadaver training, however, can be justified and be cost-effective in advanced laparoscopic training, as there is no better alternative for high fidelity simulation.

Cadaver laboratories require very specialist skills among staff looking after the specimens and the environment. There are two cadaveric processing techniques: cryopreservation (fresh frozen) and embalming (Thiel method). The traditional formalin-fixed cadavers, are not suitable for simulated surgery.

There is some evidence to indicate that fresh frozen cadavers are more favourable for laparoscopic dissection compared to classical cadaver embalming [9]. Traditionally formalin-fixed cadavers are less useful because the fixation causes tissue rigidity, loss of tissue texture, colour and consistency, limited preservation of surgical planes, and spaces, and difficulty in identifying small structures such as autonomic nerves [10]. The embalmed bodies retain more of the elastic tissue structure, which is completely different from the traditional formalin-fixed cadavers. This results in well- preserved organs and tissues with regard to colour, consistency, flexibility and plasticity [11, 12].

The environment for fresh frozen and embalmed cadavers involves storage in licenced premises and must fulfill the regulations of the Human Tissue Act in the UK [13]. This also involves proper care of donated cadavers for training, as well as security and confidentiality.

Cadavers are frozen within a week of procurement and then thawed at room temperature approximately 3 days prior to use for a training session. The cadaver

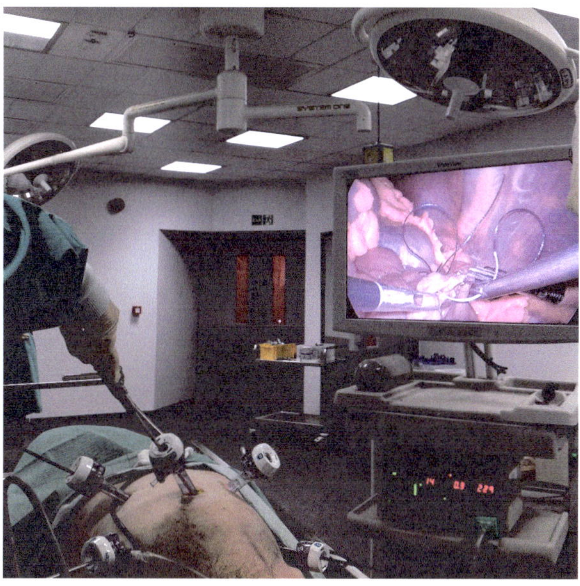

Fig. 1.2 Cadaver training model for laparoscopic surgery (with permission from the Vesalius Clinical Training Centre, Bristol)

room can be set up as an OR, with laparoscopic stacks, monitors and surgical instruments provided. Disposal of the cadaveric tissues must also be in line with national regulations or the Human Tissue Act.

Figure 1.2: Cadaver training model for laparoscopic surgery (with permission from the Vesalius Clinical Training Centre, Bristol)

Setting Up a Training Centre

It is important not to underestimate the planning required to set up a new training centre. Many readers may be familiar with situations where a MAS training facility has been set up by a lone enthusiast, only to founder when this individual moves on to new projects. In a recent survey to obtain a consensus from 57 international experts on the attributes of a training centre in advanced MAS; the following attributes were agreed on the order of importance [14]: (Fig. 1.3)

The expert group agreed that a minimum number of MAS courses (between 2 and 5 per year) should be delivered and that the unit should be actively training residents in MAS (with a minimum 2–5 trainees per year). There was a majority consensus (over 80 %) on the need for quality assurance of both training centres and of the courses provided.

There are many excellent guides for setting up a new business and project management, but here are the authors' recommendations with regard to setting up a training centre in MAS:

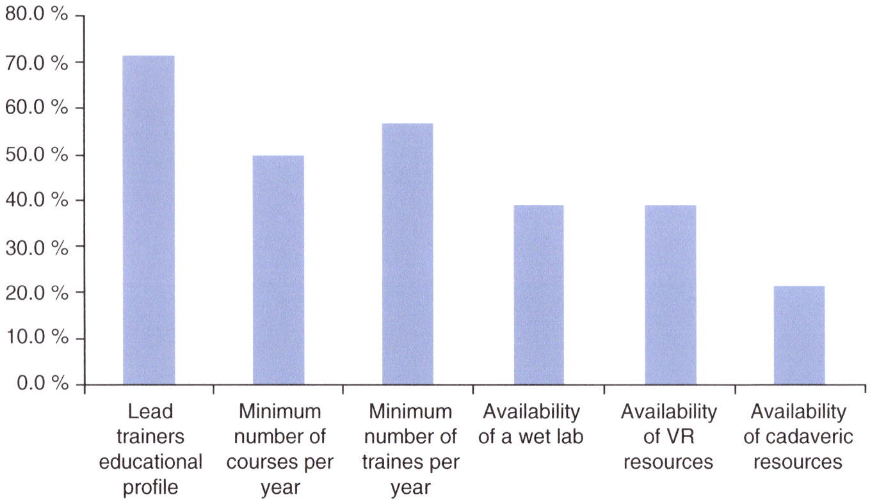

Fig. 1.3 Desirable attributes for a training centre in MAS

Ten Top Tips

1. Set up a coalition of keen surgical / clinical educators from a number of specialties.
2. Think carefully about who will need to use the centre – consider their job roles, specialties, geographical location and funding streams.
3. Look at the competition – are there any other training centres in your region/ within 50 miles? If other centres already exist, is there a way to collaborate and ensure that your own centre 'fills the gaps' in provision?
4. Which are the successful centres that you would like to emulate? – Arrange to visit them and, if possible discuss your ideas.
5. Create a business plan and get expert financial help to make sure that everything is covered.
6. Consider how you can fund the different aspects of the project: your employer, healthcare companies, grants and fundraising: – it will probably have to be a combination of all of these aspects. Think about what each group will want in return for their investment and how this will impact on what you want to achieve.
7. Still want to go ahead? Employ (or second) a good project manager to oversee the implementation of first stage of the plan – this could involve building work or re-development to create the space, procurement of equipment and hiring of staff.
8. Have a number of training activities agreed and set up to run as soon as the facility is ready – this will result in some funds coming in to the business and reassure your investors. Do not wait for the building to be completed before starting to design your training programmes.

9. Remember that each new training programme could take 6–9 months to design and could take up to 18 months to run effectively.
10. The most fantastic training centre will fail without a good team of staff to support the activities. Depending on the activity that you have planned, you will certainly need administrative and technical staff and may also want to consider academic staff or teaching fellows, together with a centre manager.

Practical Issues with Setting Up a Mas Training Centre

There are clearly some particular issues around setting up a MAS training centre [15], specifically on equipment and learning environment. Rogers et al., have summed up the requirements of a training centre focusing on the learners' need stating that "*There should be adequate facilities to accommodate the learning needs of all participants, allowing them to practice until they can demonstrate the desired level of performance…*" [16].

MAS Equipment and Industrial Support

Establishing a good relationship with industry is vital in supporting the set up and sustaining any training centre in MAS. Technology is evolving and training centres need to keep up to date with new laparoscopic equipment; such as high definition cameras and stacks, staplers and energy sources. Industry may be willing to contribute to the teaching of optimum use of their products and good liaison with them is recommended prior to delivering any educational activities. The level of support/ sponsorship from commercial companies should be discussed in the initial stages of course development to clarify their input and match the expectations. Industry can also be very useful in marketing educational events, which they sponsor through their wide network of contacts (both with surgeons and allied health care professionals). Eastablishing relationships with multiple sponsors for the educational activites is generally recommended.

Any equipment purchased must be flexible enough to meet the needs of a number of specialties and be reasonably future proof. In addition, it is vital to have the costs of maintenance contracts and depreciation of equipment included in the business plan to avoid unpleasant surprises in the future.

If you decide that VR simulations are essential, special considerations must be given to the cost of the simulators, as well as the ongoing maintenance costs. An educational curriculum needs to be in place prior to purchasing the simulators to clarify how VR will be used to assist in teaching; who will be taught on them and ensure that all learners have equal access [17]. Selection of the type of VR is based on several factors. First, VR simulation needs to fit within the training vision and the learning that the unit is providing. Secondly, if the simulation will be used as part of national courses, including assessment, it is important to align this with the local/ national regulations.

Practical Issues with Running a MAS Educational Event

Planning for Educational Events

- Think about the learners – how will they get to the training centre? Are there good public transport links? What is the parking like?
- If they come from a long distance, where can they stay overnight? Do you have a list of accommodation nearby?
- Plan other logistical issues of catering and transport from the accommodation to the training centre
- Plan course hand-outs and other educational materials to be provided to the participant, either before or when they attend the learning event.
- Consider why a potential participant will choose to come to your training centre.
- Consider your reputation, location, quality of facilities and how closely these meet their needs and value for money.

One of the most common barriers for surgeons being able to attend a training course is arranging time away from their own clinical practice, however individuals will be willing to organise this leave if the course is deemed to be of sufficient value [18].

Conducting the Educational Event

- There are generic educational resources that need to be available in any training centre:
  - audiovisual teaching resources
  - Wi-Fi and web resources
  - video production capabilities and video recording of participant activity
- For the practical skills in MAS centre:
  - adequate equipment; number of stacks per number of delegates
  - camera holders or the delegates will be assisting each other
  - adequate technical support during the course for trouble shooting and assisting the delegates when required
  - consider the working hours of the technical support team who will need to be there early to prepare for the course and to stay late to clear up.
  - allow extra time for those delegates who wish additional practice
  - Finally, ensure that you have the right faculty

Other major barriers to delivering a sustainable training programme are the availability of faculty and finances, which was highlighted in a survey of training centre managers by Kapadia et al. [19]. The financial pressures have only increased since that time, together with the increased clinical commitments on expert faculty members. Thus it is essential to build a database of enthusiastic faculty, rotate them across the training programme to prevent burn-out, and also to involve them in the development of the training programme.

Networking with Faculty of Other Training Centres

Increasingly, it may be more sensible to set up a collaborative network rather than a single training centre. Rogers et al. recognised that linking experts in different centres can provide a much more successful way to ensure that the needs of learners are met:

> As technologic innovations continue to occur, the feasibility of establishing a network of training centres should be explored. Creating this network in academic medical centres would create and excellent opportunity to study the evolving learning needs of practicing surgeons [16].

Given that most surgeons value a combination of short, intensive courses together with clinical mentorship [19], it would seem that a network of experts is best placed to provide a broad training programme. This method has been used to good effect during the National Training Programme for Laparoscopic Colorectal Surgery (LAPCO) [20], where seminars, short practical courses and long running mentorship was employed to facilitate training in laparoscopic colorectal surgery across England between 2008 and 2013.

Assessment of Educational Activities

Assessment during any educational activity is essential in training and education as it can promote learning and focus learning objectives. Assessment of the effectiveness of the education activity is also encouraged to improve the quality of the courses and to ensure the learners' needs are always met [21]. Traditionally, assessment of educational activities is performed using delegate feedback. This, however, is of limited value in refining the curriculum and ensuring the aims of the educational activities are focused. A widely-accepted model for a more structured and detailed evaluation is that of Kirkpatrick [22], who describes four levels: initial reaction of the learners' (level 1); evidence of learning as knowledge, skills or attitudes (level 2); changes in behaviour (level 3); and results in terms of structural changes undertaken by the course delegates at their home environment (level 4); or in a later refinement, evidence from trainees or course participants that their training has improved since completing the course (level 4B). A recent national training curriculum has been assessed using Kirkpatrick models to evaluate the impact of training the trainer in laparoscopic colorectal surgery and showed that the course has a direct impact on all levels, demonstrating a measurable improvement of training effectiveness [23].

Summary

The physical training environment in MAS is technology dependent and the educational environment should be a non-threatening and learner-focused to promote learning, which ultimately ensures patient's safety. Training outside the OR is influenced by the availability of simulations and their degrees of realism. VR simulations provide good training for basic MAS and cadaver training provides the optimum training for advanced MAS. There are several issues that must be considered prior to setting up a training centre, but an optimum training centre needs to provide adequate facilities to accommodate the learning needs and allow learners to practice until they can demonstrate the desired level of performance.

References

1. Larsen CR, Oestergaard J, Ottesen BS, Soerensen JL. The efficacy of virtual reality simulation training in laparoscopy: a systematic review of randomized trials. Acta Obstet Gynecol Scand. 2012;91(9):1015–28.
2. Carter F, Schijven M, Aggarwal R, Grantcharov T, Francis NK, Hanna G, Jakimowicz J. Consensus guidelines for validation of virtual reality surgical simulators: EAES Work Group for Evaluation and Implementation of Simulators and Skills Training Programmes. Surg Endosc. 2005;19(12):1523–32.
3. Carter F, Russell E, Dunkley P, Cuschieri A. Restructured animal tissue model for training in laparoscopic anti-reflux surgery. Minim Invasive Ther. 1994;3:77–80.
4. Ross GA, Christie L, McNeill A, Carter F. Novel training phantom for skills acquisition in laparoscopic nephrectomy'. Surg Endosc. 2007 (21):S148.
5. Christie L, Francis NK, Carter FJ. Tissue training model for skills acquisition for gastric bypass. Surg Endosc. 2008 (22):S36.
6. Levine RL, Kives S, Cathey G, et al. The use of lightly embalmed (fresh tissue) cadavers for resident laparoscopic training. J Minim Invasive Gynecol. 2006;13:451–6.
7. Foster JD, Gash KJ, Carter F, Longman R, Acheson A, Horgan A, Moran B, West N, Francis NK. Development and evaluation of a training curriculum for Extra-levator Abdomino Perineal Excision (ELAPE); within the LOREC National Development Programme for low rectal cancer. Colorectal dis. 2014;16(9):O308–19.
8. Corton MM, Wai CY, Babak V, et al. A compre-hensive pelvic dissection course improves obstetrics and gynecology resident proficiency in surgical anatomy. Am J Obstet Gynecol. 2003;189:647–51.
9. Tjalma WAA, Degueldre M, Van Herendael B, D'Herde K, Weyers S. Postgraduate cadaver surgery: an educational course which aims at improving surgical skills. Facts Veiw Vis ObGyn. 2013;5(1):61–5.
10. Barton DPJ, Davies DC, Mahadevan V, et al. Dissection of soft preserved cadavers in the training of gynaecological oncologists: report of the first UK workshop. Gynaecol Oncol. 2009;113:352–6.
11. Thiel W. Die Konservierung ganzer Leichen in natu¨rlichen Farben [The preservation of the whole corpse with natural color]. Ann Anat. 1992;174:185–95.
12. Thiel W. Supplement to the conservation of an entire cadaver according to W. Thiel. Ann Anat. 2002;184:267–9.

13. Human Tissue Authority. The regulator for human tissue and organs. 2004; http://www.hta.gov.uk/legislationpoliciesandcodesofpractice/legislation/humantissueact.cfm/.
14. Jervis BE, Carter FJ, Paus-Buzink S, Foster JD, Palmen R, Jakimowicz J, Francis NK. Consensus views on the optimum training curriculum for advanced laparoscopic surgery: a Delphi study. Surg Endosc. 2015 (29):S25.
15. Haluck RS, Satava RM, Fried G, Lake C, Ritter EM, Sachdeva AK, Seymour NE, Terry ML, Wilks D. Establishing a simulation center for surgical skills: what to do and how to do it. Surg Endosc. 2007;21(7):1223–32.
16. Rogers DA, Elstein AS, Bordage G. Improving continuing medical education for surgical techniques: applying the lessons learned in the first decade of minimal access surgery". Ann Surg. 2001;233(2):159–66.
17. van Dongen KW, Ahlberg G, Bonavina L, Carter FJ, Grantcharov TP, Hyltander A, Schijven MP, Stefani A, van der Zee DC, Broeders IAMJ. European consensus on a competency-based virtual reality training program for basic endoscopic surgical psychomotor skills. Surg Endosc. 2010;25(1):166–71.
18. Wallace T, Birch DW. A needs assessment study for continuing professional development in advanced minimally invasive surgery. Am J Surg. 2007;193:593–6.
19. Kapadia MR, DaRosa DA, MacRae HM, Dunnington GL. Current assessment and future directions of surgical skills laboratories. J Surg Educ. 2007;64(5):260–5.
20. Coleman MG, Hanna GB, Kennedy R. The National Training Programme for Laparoscopic Colorectal Surgery in England: a new training paradigm. Colorectal Dis. 2011;13:614–6.
21. Steinert Y, Mann K, Centeno A, et al. A systematic review of faculty development initiatives designed to improve teaching effectiveness in medical education: BEME Guide No. 8. Med Teach. 2006;28(6):497–526.
22. Kirkpatrick JD. Evaluating training programs. 3rd ed. San Francisco: Berret-Koehler Publ; 2006.
23. Mackenzie H, Cuming T, Miskovic D, et al. Design, delivery, and validation of a trainer curriculum for the national laparoscopic colorectal training program in England. Ann Surg. 2015;261(1):149–56.

Chapter 2
Training Curriculum in Minimal Access Surgery

J.J. Jakimowicz and Sonja Buzink

Introduction

Historically, the term 'curriculum' was originally related to the concept of a course of studies followed by a pupil in a teaching institution. In recent decades, however the concept of curriculum has evolved and gained in importance to the extent that it may overlap with another terminology; epistemology (i.e., the concept being used to indicate all dimensions of the educational process, without allowing any differentiated analytical approach to its complexity).

A curriculum is far more than just a syllabus or training course programme; it outlines the template and model enabling and enhancing the process of learning and skills acquisition. It defines what has to be taught and learned in terms of knowledge and skill and it indicates teaching, learning and assessment methodology. Moreover, it contains recommendations of suitable and validated learning and training modalities enabling effective delivery and implementation of the program in practice. In order to become a formal curriculum the program has to be put in written form and be published [1, 2].

This chapter focuses on curriculum design for minimal access surgery (MAS) and other image-based procedures, specifically for surgeons in training and consultant surgeons wishing to start laparoscopic surgery practice.

J.J. Jakimowicz, MD, PhD, FRCS, Ed (✉)
Research and Education, Catharina Hospital,
Michelangelolaan 2, Eindhoven 5623 EJ, The Netherlands
e-mail: jakimowi@planet.nl

S. Buzink
Faculty of Industrial Design Engineering, Delft University of Technology,
Landbergstraat 15, Delft 2628 CE, The Netherlands
e-mail: sonjabuzink@yahoo.com

N. Francis et al. (eds.), *Training in Minimal Access Surgery*,
DOI 10.1007/978-1-4471-6494-4_2

Throughout time a number of curricula for training in MAS were developed, described and evaluated. Most of these focussed on the VR-simulation as a main component, specifically for training basic laparoscopic surgery, and grossly focussed on acquisition of skills. Some of them lacked a cognitive teaching component as well as an adequate assessment of knowledge and skills of trainees acquired during training [3, 4].

The Fundamental of Laparoscopic Surgery (FLS) was developed by the Society of American Gastrointestinal and Endoscopic Surgeons (SAGES) and is one of the most well known curricula. A considerable number of publications as well as data regarding evaluation of FLS are available. The FLS program consists of both skills and cognitive training. Controlled randomised trials provide evidence of transfer of skills acquired during the FLS program to the operating room (OR) [5]. However, it has to be realised that FLS is limited to training basic components of laparoscopic skills and lacks procedural components [6].

Models of Curricula

Recently Cristancho et al. 2011 [7] proposed a framework-based approach to the design of simulation-augmented surgical education and training programs. First of all, authors warned designers of educational and training curricula of the potential pitfalls in the process of developing a curriculum. These are a lack of: (i) an objective identification of training needs, (ii) a structured assessment of performance, (iii) a systematic design methodology and finally (iv) a research centred evaluation. A detailed description of the process of designing a surgical simulation has been published by Cristancho et al. in 2011 [7] and describes an augmented training, consisting of three sequential steps: (i) aim, (ii) fine tune- and (iii) follow through.

1. Aim

   The first step is focused on the selection of tasks or skills to be taught. Subsequently the procedure is broken down into tasks, subtasks and individual skills. The design mapping stage enables identification of specific skills to be simulated. At this stage of development of a curriculum the criteria for evaluating simulations as defined by Kneebone [8] may be considered and used. Simulation should: (1) allow for sustained deliberate practice within a safe environment, allowing consolidation of skills acquired within a curriculum assuming regular enforcement be supported by easy access/presence of experts for as long as needed. (2) map on to real life clinical experience and be supportive of actual practice. (3) provide supportive motivation and learner-centred environment, constructive to the learning process.

   The authors propose the use of the Motor and Cognitive Modelling Diagram (MCMD), a general task-modelling tool developed for this purpose [9]. MCMD can be used for mapping the steps of any surgical procedure. It allows the recording and analysis of ideal sequences, selected by surgeons during various procedures [7].

2. The fine tuning

   This is a verification stage involving development of additional mapping for more experts to validate the work and process them into flow diagrams. The use of the Delphi-technique should be considered to achieve consensus of a panel of experts, allowing identification of training and simulation techniques as well as allowing choice of teaching methodology.
3. Follow through

   This is the final stage of proposed process and consists of implementation and validation of developed simulation content and scenarios.

Framework of Curricula

Aggarwal et al. proposed a framework for development of a curriculum recommending five steps [10]:

(a) knowledge-based learning
(b) deconstruction of the procedure into component tasks
(c) training in a skills laboratory environment
(d) demonstration of transfer of skills to the real environment
(e) granting of privileges for independent practice

The authors of this framework for systematic training and assessment of technical skills claim that it is simplistic, feasible and generic to any branch of medicine that involves acquisition of a technical skill. They conclude that the model also provides an opportunity to develop a valid, objective and viable method to assess technical skills both in laboratory-based and real environments [10].

The formula for a successful laparoscopic skills curriculum elaborated by Stefanidis and Heniford combines didactic sessions with manual skills training on a simulator allowing trainees to gain knowledge to improve their understanding of the tasks and procedures [11].

It is expected that direct application of knowledge into practise may improve the retention of information compared to didactic teaching alone. The suggested simulator-based curriculum for cognitive and manual skills training in one academic year starts with initiative ability testing and baseline assessment of skills. Task demonstrations, video tutorials and deliberate practise in a number of distributed sessions (up to ten) follow until the training goal/proficiency is achieved. During these sessions adequate continuous feedback is of importance. Distributed sessions are meant to safeguard retention of acquired skills [12]. After achieving the training goal/proficiency over the training period/sessions it is recommended that this be followed by maintenance training. Maintenance training is an important element of the process and is scheduled as testing/training sessions every 1–3 months after initial proficiency is achieved. The post-training assessment follows after maintenance training is accomplished. Testing at the start (baseline) and at the end of the curriculum, combined with performance monitoring during training, may help to boost trainees motivation by enabling them to track improvements in their performance as stated by Fried [13].

Successful laparoscopic skills curriculum depends on many factors including participants' motivations, available resources and personal training and facility commitment. Kern et al. [14] described curriculum development for medical education as a six-step approach as early as in 1998. Steps include: performing a general need assessment, developing rational target's needs, defining goals and objectives, selecting adequate evaluation criteria and finally performing a program of evaluation and feedback.

The process of curriculum planning and development extensively elaborated by Hardan should be considered in ten steps [15]:

1. identifying the need,
2. establishing the learning outcomes,
3. agreeing the content,
4. organising the content,
5. deciding g the educational strategy,
6. deciding the teaching methods,
7. preparing the assessment,
8. communication about curriculum,
9. the educational environment
10. management of the curriculum.

These steps, reviewed in the context of trends of medical by Hardan, are applicable and may be used as a guideline for planning and development of training curricula in MAS [15].

Key Elements and Essential Factors for Successful Delivery of Educational and Training Curricula

The development of a training program in general and specifically for training in MAS cannot be left to chance. It has to be prepared and elaborated in a structured way, taking into account not only basic educational rules but also current trends in medical education and training of health providers.

Deliberate Practice

Deliberate practise is essential for acquisition of skills and performance improvement. It is a form of training, based upon focused repetitive practice during which a trainee monitors his/her performance, corrects errors and receives adequate feedback, which supports the achievement of steady and consistent improvement of performance [16, 17].

Motivation, Internal and External

Motivation, particularly the internal one, remains the true driving force for the learner/trainee to achieve the goals of a program of training. It is unique for the trainee and strongly dependent on personality traits, and is thus difficult to change. The role model behaviour of the trainer is of particular importance in driving motivation and enthusiasm among trainees. External motivation may influence and even alter the attitude and behaviour of trainees in order to truly become involved in the process and pursue the desired outcomes. Several external factors may positively influençe trainees. For simulation-based training factors such as adequate computer-based VR-procedural simulation with haptic feedback, appealing tissue models, surgery upon live animals, video tutorials and many other measures should be considered.

Stefanidis et al. recently reported on the role of simulator performance goals to boost motivation of trainees as well as skills laboratory attendance [18]. The study showed that use of optional goals in addition to standard proficiency levels results in improved trainee participation and motivation to practice and attendance at the skills laboratory. Moreover, a safe skills laboratory environment and healthy competition in simulation-based training with adequate feedback is an important stimulus. Mandatory participation in a training course or curriculum however remains the most effective external measure.

In the past, most of the European countries had external demotivating factors such as long working hours, limited free time, overload of clinical work, which with-held trainees from simulation-based training. With the reduced working hours as a result of the European Working Time Directive (EWTD) this nowadays plays a secondary role.

Performance Feedback

Technical skills feedback can be defined as providing essential information regarding performance of tasks of the procedure to the trainee in course of a performance itself [19]. Intrinsic feedback consists of performance-related information, available directly during performance as visual, auditory information or haptic perception. Recent papers indicate potential benefit of haptic feedback on skills acquisition during VR-simulation training [20]. In spite of improvements to the haptics of VR-simulators the discussion on the precise value of haptics is ongoing. However, trainees seem to be more motivated when working with simulators providing some haptic feedback.

Extrinsic or augmented feedback consists of information provided to the trainee by an external source, and enhances intrinsic feedback, resulting in an improvement in performance. As stated by Magil, extrinsic feedback facilitates the achievement of skills and motivates the learner to continue to work towards the achievement of skills [19]. There is no doubt that providing augmented feedback versus no feedback at all results in better skill acquisition and retention. There are a number of studies that provide strong evidence on the possible impact and value of the external feedback during simulator training, resulting in improved skills acquisition [12, 21, 22].

Extrinsic feedback can be provided to trainees in two different forms: formative or summative feedback. Formative feedback is provided during active performance of the task or procedure, correcting errors and therefore influencing the performance. Its intensity, duration and frequency may vary depending on the expertise and skills of both the trainee and the trainer. Summative feedback is focused at the end of the task or procedure performance and applies equally to multiple choice examinations, scenario-based examinations and problem-based tests. The frequency of feedback should be intense, almost 100 % [23] In our opinion extrinsic feedback should be provided during all modules and modalities and skills training but not be exaggerated.

Regarding instructor feedback, it is often presumed that the role of instructor feedback in procedural training using VR-simulation is limited. A randomised prospective trial on instructor feedback versus no instructor feedback showed exactly the opposite effect. Instructor feedback increases efficiency when training complex operational, procedural tasks on VR-simulator. Time and repetitions used to achieve a predefined proficiency level were significantly shorter in the group that received instructor feedback compared with the control group [24].

One has to realise that inappropriate feedback may result in a negative effect on skills acquisition. To avoid risks related to inappropriate feedback, trainers should provide the feedback in a standardised and uniform manner.

Effective Task Demonstration

Comprehensive detailed, standardised, well-structured instruction and demonstration plays a paramount role in supporting task/procedure performance and is crucial for acquisition of technical skills. It helps trainees to understand the tasks or procedures and in planning the best approach by enabling them to create a suitable mental model of how to successfully accomplish a task or procedure. The most frequently used instruction method is demonstration of a task by an expert or trainer supported by verbal information. However, video-based instruction using CD-ROM-recordings appears useful and effective when applied in the context of VR-simulation, and has proven to enhance the acquisition of technical skills [25]. The role of video-based educational information when training technical skills on animal tissue models or in life animal should not be underestimated. This provides important and additional information on the anatomy of the animal or animal tissue model, clarifies the component tasks and provides standardised guidance on how to accomplish the task/procedure. Providing multiple and sometimes contradictory manner feedback to accomplish the taks or procedure can thus be avoided. Video tutorials should be provided well before the training. It has been demonstrated that such an approach is superior to provision of the tutorial just before the training session starts [26].

Practice Distribution

In most MAS training curricula, training takes place in 1 or 2 days of mass practise. A successful MAS curriculum provides trainees with the opportunity to master tasks and acquire skills in several training sessions with periods of rest between sessions (so called distributed practice). Research has shown that distributed practice is superior to mass practice for skills acquisition in simulation training [27–29]. The benefit of distributed practice is presumably a result of learning during the rest periods between training sessions. The explanation of this phenomenon is the assumption that practice activates neural processes in the brain that continue to evolve many hours after training sessions [30]. Training sessions that evoke changes in brain activity possibly initiates long-term effects enhancing consolidation of the initial practice/learning experience. In spite of the benefits of practice distribution a number of issues have to be addressed. Controversy exists regarding inter-training intervals and numbers of sessions. It is doubtful if optimal practise distribution and training intervals can be established at all, not only due to task specific dependency of skills acquisition but mainly other factors such as pre-existing experience, knowledge, initiative abilities and the psychological profile of the trainee. Moreover, the training environment may play an important role as well. If the program is not restricted to one hospital or institution the trainee will face major problems such as time restrictions and availability of trainee to practice. The logistics of a program for trainees coming from different areas of a country or from abroad remains a major obstacle because of inherent geographic variations.

Proficiency-Based Training

The traditional approach to training entailed time-based curricula with a pre-determined, time duration of training (or repetitive-based practice with a pre-set number of training episodes of task repetition) before training is considered to be completed. However, this model does not take into account factors such as prior experience, baseline skills, personal abilities or attitude and motivation of the trainee, all of which are critical for the acquisition of skills. Such a curriculum may result in under- or overtraining and is thus less effective and certainly less efficient.

On the contrary, proficiency-based curricula are based upon clearly defined training endpoints or goals, derived from expert performance and indicate a clear target for the trainee to achieve during training. Proficiency-based training gives trainees an opportunity to review their results and to set new performance targets after completion or execution of each training session. Feedback on performance is provided, motivation stimulated, deliberate practice promoted (reinforced) leading to enhanced skills acquisition [20, 31]. Many researchers have stated that proficiency-based training is superior to time duration or repetition-based training [5, 14, 32–35]. Our own study confirms these findings and underlines the benefits of proficiency-based training [36].

We believe that a proficiency-based approach to training should not be restricted to simulator training, but is also applicable to simulation training in general, independent of the modality used. Its use for procedural training in surgery and impact on performance is worth considering as a subject for further research.

Task Difficulty and Practice Variability

Practice variability and progressively increasing task difficulty are of importance in the process of developing a curriculum. A well-structured technical skills training program provides practice variability as well as the opportunity to train with a progressively increasing level of task complexity. The influence of this factor on skills acquisition is well-documented [37, 38]. Whereas block practice refers to preset, specified selected tasks, practice variability allows repetition of the same task at random, which appears to be advantageous [39, 40]. It is however dependent on the complexity of the task [41]. Increasing the complexity or difficulty of tasks, especially when using simulator training, results in enhanced skills acquisition [37]. One may presume that using this method, whatever simulation modality is used, would enrich the curriculum [4].

Simulation-based training recommended by most educators, takes place in the "safe" setting of a skills laboratory. Studies often indicate that transfer of the acquired skill to real operating room setting benefits by this approach. However, more recent results of systematic reviews on the role of disturbance and interference during training show that training in settings resembling the real OR enhances transfer of skills acquired in the "safe" laboratory setting. From our own studies we conclude that simulation training in a setting with an increased cognitive load, the presence of disruptions and interference, and thus "out of the bubble", improves the transfer of skills [42, 43]. The overwhelming majority of studies on simulation training in a skills laboratory setting do not pay attention to the importance of the physical aspects of the skills laboratory environment. Most skills laboratories do not comply with the ergonomic principles and settings for MAS. Trainees may possess some theoretical knowledge of ergonomics of MAS in the OR, but do not have the opportunity to learn and practise this in the skills laboratory in order to transfer it to the OR [44].

Assessment and Choosing the Method of Assessment

The role of assessment is to measure performance, which can be used effectively as feedback for the main aspects of a curriculum. It allows a measurement of a trainee's level of performance and provides an indication of effectiveness and measures appropriateness of the course content. A wide range of assessment tools is available to be applied in the framework of simulation-based curricula. It is important to choose and define an adequate assessment method, keeping in mind when and what assessment should take place. The assessment tool has to be feasible, valid and reliable.

It is worth however, defining validity prior to exploring the different assessment methods: Validity is defined as 'the property of being true, correct and in conformity with reality [45]; subdivided into different levels (validity of tests):

(i) Face validity addresses users' opinion about the functionality and realism
(ii) Content validity: content is suited to measure what it is supposed to measure
(iii) Construct validity: measures the trait it is supposed to measure
(iv) Discriminant validity (variant of construct validity): discriminates between different experts
(v) Concurrent validity: compares to a standard/another test measuring the same trait
(vi) Predictive validity: extent of prediction of future performance

Assessment Tools/Methods, Applicable for Performance Assessment During Training Curricula

Assessment of performance on simulators is mostly by the use of metrics for task duration and error rate. These very basic parameters are often supported by additional performance metrics such as trajectory, velocity and economy of movements. These criteria, however, may provide a misleading picture of a trainee's readiness to perform in a clinical setting. The influence of the demanding and stressful environment of the OR must not be underestimated [46]. Using complementary psycho-physiological measurements to estimate cognitive load and stress level may contribute to performance assessment and may augment skills acquisition and transfer [43].

Assessments based on observational tools are applicable and useful for both skills laboratories and work place settings. These tools allow identification of specific sets of deficient skills, and provide an opportunity for formative and summative feedback during task performance. Direct observation of technical skills throughout different stages of a curriculum is critical for the assessment of skills acquisition by the trainee [47]. There are three main categories of observational tools: rating scales for the assessment of generic skills, procedure-specific skills assessment and a combination of generic and procedure-specific skills assessment [48].

Rating Scales for Assessment of Generic Skills

For evaluation of generic skills the Global Rating Scale (GRS) appears to be effective in term of feasibility, face validity, content validity, and construct validity as shown in different studies [48, 49]. The GRS shows a high acceptability and good construct validity on a low-cost high fidelity porcine model, used for surgical skills assessment, as reported by Leong et al. [50].

Another effective system is the McGill Inanimate System for Training and Evaluation of Laparoscopic Skills, consisting of five tasks that are evaluated by measuring the time to completion and accuracy. It is validated and reliable for assessment of the generic skills of trainees and applied to the development of Fundamentals in Laparoscopic Surgery (FLS program). Finally, the Global Operative Assessment of Laparoscopic Skills (GOALS) assessment tool was studied and validated for procedures as cholecystectomy and appendectomy. It is reported to be feasible, reliable and superior to a task checklist for evaluation of technical skills [51–54].

Procedure-Specific Skills Assessment

For procedure-specific skills assessment, the Observational Clinical Human Reliability Analysis (OCHRA) uses error analysis adopted from human reliability methods [51–54]. Tang et al. reported a task analysis for assessment of cognitive and technical skills using OCHRA during laparoscopic cholecystectomy [52]. It has also been used for analysis of errors enacted by surgical trainees during skills courses. Different studies showed content and construct validity of the tool in both the clinical and skills laboratory setting [53, 54].

A large number of procedure-specific checklists have been developed and reported to be feasible, valid and reliable for different levels of training [48]. The Global Assessment of Gastrointestinal Endoscopic Skills (GAGES) s one of the checklists and has shown to be valid and reliable for assessment of trainees [55]. GAGES upper endoscopy (UE) and colonoscopy (C) are 5-point Likert rating scales developed by expert endoscopists. For UE, domains assessed were esophageal intubation, scope navigation, maintenance of a clear field, instrumentation (when biopsy, injection or polypectomy were performed), and overall quality of the examination; for C, these were scope navigation, strategies for scope advancement, clear field, instrumentation (when performed), and overall quality [55].

Combination of Procedure-Specific and Generic Tools

Objective Structured Assessment of Technical Skills (OSATS) consists of two parts: assessment of procedural skills and assessment of generic skills, including the judgement of knowledge and handling of instruments. Many studies have been carried out to validate OSATS, mostly in a skills laboratory setting. OSATS have high face validity and strong construct validity with significant correlation between surgical performance scores and level of experience [56].

The Global Assessment of Skills (GAS) tool has been developed and was validated at Imperial College for the English national training program in laparoscopic colorectal surgery (LAPCO). It showed a high reliability and significant construct validity. The GAS tool is also available for procedures as cholecystectomy and appendectomy, and is used within the laparoscopic surgical skills program.

The Competency Assessment Tool (CAT) was developed and implemented to evaluate technical surgical performance in the LAPCO program and showed construct validity and was reliable in demonstrating differences in levels of competency [57]. CAT was modified and developed as an assessment tool for cholecystectomy and appendectomy, and applied for assessment of trainees in the Laparoscopic Surgical Skills (LSS) curriculum.

Self Assessment

Medical professional societies consider self-assessment a reflection of an individual's own performance to be a safe regulation and self-monitoring aspect of the lifelong performance of a medical specialist. Life-long learning requires that healthcare providers are able not only to work independently, but also to assess their own performance and their own progress adequately [58]. The main components of self-assessment are: (i)review and evaluation of their own performance using pre-set criteria, (ii) explain the processes used and (iii) identify their own strengths and weaknesses. To be able to self-assess trainees should possess a set of criteria developed for performance in their specific domain, which are already known by trainees in advance as a gold standard for comparison.

Self-assessment is nowadays frequently used in the course of simulation training, as well as in the work place. It is presumed to benefit simulation-based training, not only by the faculty but because it is self-driven, it reduces the need for supervision and results in lower program costs [58, 59]. Poor correlation between self-assessment and assessment by experts has been reported in individual studies and confirmed by a meta-analysis of studies in higher education [60, 61]. However, there is also research showing a high correlation between the two, indicating the usefulness of self-assessment. In a study on self-assessment of technical and non-technical skills in high fidelity simulation Arora et al. found that surgeons are capable of self-assessing their technical skills regardless of their experience, but not necessarily their non-technical skills [62]. This confirms other reports as suggesting that Junior surgeons overestimate their communication and teamwork abilities, while senior surgeons underestimate their non-technical skills [63]. One should not forget that simulation-based training provides the opportunity for formative feedback, when comparing the outcomes with one of the supervising experts.

Monitoring and Evaluation of Curricula

Monitoring

Developing a successful training and educational curriculum in MAS is a complex, dynamic and evolving process. Continuous monitoring and evaluating of the curriculum is mandatory to respond adequately to the ongoing changes in surgical techniques, new technology, new simulation and training modalities, and trends in medical education. Basic issues to be monitored are: (1) Are the criteria for candidate selection correct? (2) Do the participants meet the selection criteria for respective level of the training program? (3) Are trainers available, motivated and do they have the capacity to teach, supervise and assess? (4) Is there a need for a specific 'train the trainer' program? (5) Are there qualified technical skills laboratory staff available to facilitate the training?

With regard to training and learning the following aspects are of importance: (1) Is the syllabus/knowledge package adequate and updated? (2) Is the curriculum as outlined effective in practice? (3) Is the balance between the different training/learning components appropriate in regard to the desired outcomes of the training? (4) Are e-learning, online MCQ and scenario-based examinations, video tutorials available, and adequate? (5) Are the simulation models and modalities validated and available? (6) Are the skills laboratory facilities appropriate and if not, what changes are necessary? (7) Are assessment methods adequate to assess skills and knowledge? (8) Are the assessment tools of the appropriate level, reliable and valid?

Finally, with regard to training resources, are the performance standards, benchmarks and different levels of training achieved? [64]

Monitoring should enable identification of serious setbacks or bottle-necks in the course of the implementation of the curriculum and ongoing monitoring should safeguard achievement of the expected outcomes.

There are several approaches to monitoring the curriculum. One is by observation, preferably carried out by an independent reviewer. However, even if the information is collected in a standardised way, it may be prone to observer bias. Feedback questionnaires can, if well-structured and containing questions relevant for fine-tuning of the curriculum, provide a huge amount of information. It should be a regular practice to anonymously collect these kinds of questionnaires. 69]

Structured or semi-structured meetings of the Curriculum Committee are a platform for reviewing information the whole curriculum or elements of it. The outcome of such meetings should result in actions to improve the curriculum.

Finally, the results of the trainee's assessments are an important element of the monitoring process. Analysis of formative and summative assessments may indicate if they are adequately performed and reliable. Moreover, they can show if present training goals are being achieved.

Evaluation

Adequate evaluation of a curriculum provides information regarding its quality for stakeholders, trainees, educators, trainers and management. The reasons for evaluation are estimation of the quality of the program, detection of shortcomings, review of potential improvements, assurance of achieved pre-set endpoints, analysis of cost-effectiveness and assessment of the fulfilment of the needs of trainees and other stakeholders.

When evaluating a curriculum the following should be considered: (1) Are the objectives realistic and relevant to the current state of MAS? (2) Is the target group of trainees well-defined and do trainees fulfil the entry requirements for the level of training offered? (3) Are the syllabus and recommended reading materials well-matched to the level of training at each part of the program (4) Are the training modalities/multimodality simulators (box trainers, augmented reality), VR-simulators adequately validated and available? (5) Is the balance of technical skills training, case discussion, didactic lectures and assessment appropriate? (6) Are the logistics of the curriculum adequate to allow formative and summative feedback? (7) Do trainers possess the skills needed to deliver the curriculum? (8) Is the training environment adequate and up to current standards? [65]

The Laparoscopic Surgical Skills (LSS) Program

A first and crucial step in considering development of the LSS program was the identification of the need for such a curriculum. Dunn described the following steps to identify curriculum needs: the wise men approach of consultation with stakeholders, the study of errors in practise, clinical incidents studies and the study of star performers [65]. Opinions of experts, educators, "wise men" in MAS were the driving power in development of the LSS curriculum and assessment program [66, 67].

In the USA the Accreditation Council of Graduate Medical Education (ACGME) and the American Board of Medical Specialities (ABMS) identified six general core competences in the USA. Core competencies in laparo-endoscopic surgery are: (1) preoperative care: diagnosis, preoperative preparation and judgement (2) operative performance: integrated cognitive skills, technical skills and judgement (3) postoperative care: monitoring, treatment and judgement [68]. To acquire and assess these competences the need for structured training and education is obvious.

The introduction of the European Work Time Directive (EWTD) in Europe, resulting in limited exposure of trainees to clinical work and a restricted number of cases operated under supervision, forced training program directors to create opportunities for skills lab training in MAS. Reports on adverse results in MAS procedures turned the attention of patients and the media to the risks related to MAS and other image-based procedures. Health care authorities in some countries, such as the Netherlands, issued recommendations urging development and implementation of training for MAS. These factors contributed to the development of the LSS program. Nowadays the importance of training and education in new technology-dependent surgical techniques is recognised widely by stakeholders, patients, surgical societies, the media and governmental bodies.

The LSS program, an initiative of the European Association of Endoscopic Surgery (EAES), is the most recently developed curriculum and comprehensive performance assessment program. In order to develop, implement, promote and evaluate this program the Laparoscopic Surgical Skills Foundation was created

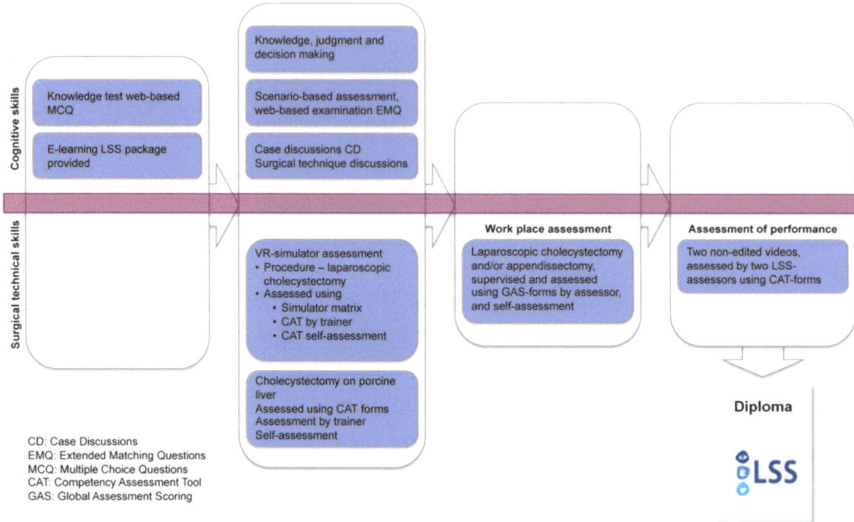

Fig. 2.1 Laparoscopic Surgical Skills LSS curriculum and assessment program

(www.lss-surgical.eu). The curriculum and assessment standards are the result of a close cooperation between experts in MAS, members of the EAES and the Faculty of Design Engineering at the Delft University of Technology, Six PhD candidates contributed to the content, structure, monitoring and evaluation of the different elements of the LSS-program [69]. The LSS-curriculum and assessment program focuses on safeguarding the quality of performance in MAS surgery, and goes far beyond the basic skills. This is achieved by combining an assessment of knowledge, judgement and decision-making in the skills laboratory and by multiple choice online examinations and scenario-based examinations with work place clinical assessment of performance on the indicated procedures (Fig. 2.1).

It should be stressed that LSS is first and, by far, the most developed tool to offer a standard for comprehensive performance assessment. However, for such a standard to become meaningful it should become fully integrated as a part of training curriculum for surgery and part of training and education in MAS. LSS provides recommendations for multimodality simulation training, validated assessments, a syllabus of selected reading lists for speciality surgery, as well as the assessment by online patient-based discussions, multiple choice and scenario-based assessment examinations.

Assessment tools, such as CAT and GAS assessment forms, for use in skills laboratory and clinical settings are available and should be used during core events of the program in the LSS accredited centre. Accreditation acts as a warranty for appropriate level of training and assessment. Only when the content and standards of the curriculum are met can a prospective centre become an EAES/ LSS accredited centre and participate in the LSS program. To provide the upmost value for the trainees it is of paramount importance that centres running the LSS-program apply

Table 2.1 Laparoscopic Surgical Skills (LSS) Grades

Grade 1		Grade 2
Level 1	Level 2 – advanced procedures	Speciality surgery
Elementary laparoscopic skills	Suturing & Dissection + energized instruments	Separate assessments & courses:
Basic knowledge & skills Index procedures Cholecystectomie Appendicectomy Diagnostic laparoscopy	Index procedures: Anti-reflux procedures Incisional hernia repair Inguinal hernia repair Perforated duodenal ulcer Common bile duct exploration Splenectomy Parastomal hernia repair Difficult cholecystectomy	Colon surgery Bariatric surgery Robotic surgery Hepatobiliary

for endorsement by their local/national bodies, such as surgical societies or national accreditation bodies. At present there is no single organisation to offer pan-European approval.

The Program Outline

The design of the LSS-program is based on key elements and factors, the model curriculum discussed in this chapter, as well as the elements and factors, essential for delivery and successful implementation of the curriculum.

The LSS-program is developed for surgeons in training, surgical fellows and practising surgeons wanting to start their laparoscopic surgery practice. The program is constructed around two grades and different levels to attend the divergent needs of surgeons of different levels of training or surgical expertise. In addition, eligible candidates are offered an option to enrol either to the LSS-assessment solely, or for LSS accredited course in which the LSS-assessment is embedded. The basic laparoscopic skills and the basic laparoscopic procedures are embedded in level I, while the advanced laparoscopic procedures are covered by the level II of Grade I. Grade II consists of a curriculum and assessment, focused on speciality surgery. Each level within the LSS-program addresses specific index procedures. An overview of LSS-grades and levels is presented in Table 2.1. The focus of the program is quality of performance of laparoscopic procedures and not just abstract tasks.

Comprehensive Assessment of Laparoscopic Skills

LSS offers a standard for comprehensive performance assessment for training and education in laparoscopic surgery. To obtain the LSS-diploma participating surgeons need to pass several types of assessment to assure that they have reached the

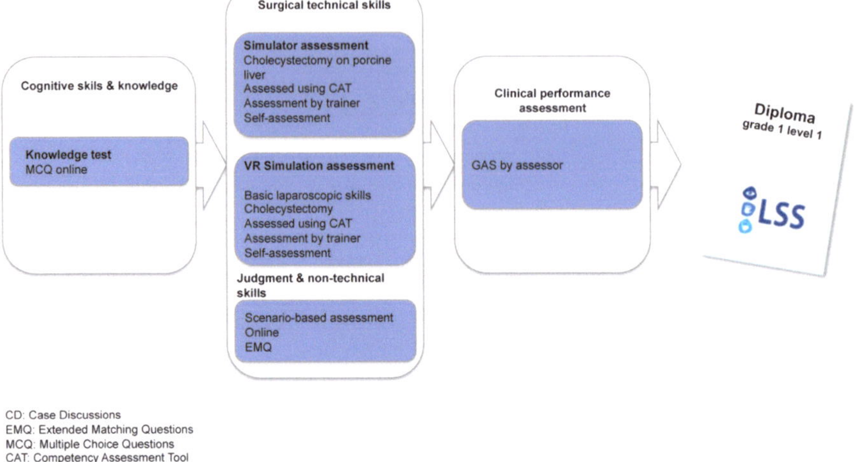

Fig. 2.2 Laparoscopic Surgical Skills LSS curriculum. Structure of comprehensive assessment

appropriate level of performance (Fig. 2.2). Within this series of assessments the proficiency of surgeons in cognitive skills, surgical technical skills, judgment and decision-making is evaluated.

Adequate knowledge of the theory of basic laparoscopic and procedure-specific topics (e.g., techniques, instrumentation, energised instruments and ergonomics) corresponding to the LSS-level entered is tested using a web-based knowledge test. To prepare for this test all participants who enrol for LSS are provided online with a set of course documents describing theory and knowledge on the relevant index procedures. This applies for trainees, certified surgeons, both those who enrol only in the assessment process, as well as those who enrol for the accredited course. This is to ensure that the potential local preferences to which surgeons can be habituated will not impede performance during the assessment. The course documents are, as far as possible, based on a general international consensus on the indicator procedures and the training of laparoscopic skills. Since the available general consensus on theory is still limited, international renowned experts on laparoscopic surgery were consulted to establish the content by means of modified Delphi surveys. Passing the knowledge test is an admission requirement for the course and the scenario-based assessment and simulation assessment.

The aim of the simulator assessment is to certify that a sufficient level of psychomotor and technical surgical skills has been achieved to start performing the specific index procedures on patients under supervision of the mentor/trainer. The focus of all LSS-assessments is primarily on procedural knowledge and skills; however possession of basic laparoscopic skills is essential before mastering any procedural skills. For this reason simulator assessments of LSS-level also comprise some tasks to evaluate basic skills. Participants need to reliably demonstrate adequate performance of a selection of basic and procedural tasks on the assessment simulators to pass the simulator assessment successfully. The simulator assessment is an admission requirement for the clinical performance assessment.

Performance of a laparoscopic cholecystectomy on a porcine liver is assessed using the CAT forms. The same applies to the procedural simulation, while the performance on the VR procedural simulator is by metrics of the system and also using the CAT-forms. Self-assessment and assessment by the tutor takes place in both settings and is used for the formative and summative assessment.

To facilitate criterion-based training benchmarks have been established throughout the program. Pass/fail benchmarks are re-established in the scores of the participants, who performed the LSS-simulator assessment within the first LSS-year. We purposely chose the use of performance scores of the target group and not the scores of experts. This logically follows from the objectives of the assessment and is also based on our previous experience with performance of both surgical trainees and laparoscopic experts on surgical VR-simulator.

The hands-on training in LSS courses is criterion-based. The training benchmarks in LSS accredited courses are set as a challenging, yet realistically achievable level to keep all participants motivated. The performance parameters provided by the simulators throughout the training provide the participants and trainers direct feedback on milestone achievements. Participants, who succeed in achieving the training benchmarks within the course, can expect to pass the simulator assessment easily.

Having passed the scenario-based examination and simulation assessment a trainee has proven that a sufficient level of knowledge, psychometric and technical skills have been achieved to start performing specific index procedures under supervision of a mentor at their respective hospital. The workplace assessment takes place under supervision of a mentor/experienced laparoscopic surgeon at the hospital where the trainee works. For the purpose of assessment and feedback GAS forms are used.

Having collected a sufficient number of points participants of the program have to provide two non-edited videos of index procedures for assessment by two independent LSS assessors. At this point the trainee receives a diploma that indicates he/she fulfilled the requirements of the respective level of LSS program. In case of Grade I-level I the trainee is up to a standard that should enable them to perform index procedures, while the decision to allow the trainee to perform these procedures independently is the responsibility of the local training program director/mentor. Preliminary experience with LSS curriculum grade 1, level 1, has been recently published [70, 71].

References

1. Dent J, Harden MR. A practical guide for medical teachers. Edinburgh/New York: Elsevier Health Sciences UK; 2009.
2. McKimm J1, Barrow M. Curriculum and course design. Br J Hosp Med (Lond). 2009;70(12):714–7.

3. Schijven MP, Jakimowicz JJ, Broeders IA, Tseng LN. The Eindhoven laparoscopic cholecystectomy training course – improving operating room performance using virtual reality training: results from the First EAES accredited virtual reality training curriculum. Surg Endosc. 2005;19(9):1220–6.
4. Aggarwal R, Grantcharov T, Moorthy K, et al. A competency-based virtual reality training curriculum for the acquisition of laparoscopic psychomotor skill. Am J Surg. 2006;191(1): 128–33.
5. Sroka G, Feldman LS, Vassilou MC, et al. Fundamentals of laparoscopic surgery simulator training to proficiency improves laparoscopic performance in the operating room- a randomzed controlled trial. Am J Surg. 2010;199:115–20.
6. Ritter EM1, Scott DJ. Design of a proficiency-based skills training curriculum for the fundamentals of laparoscopic surgery. Surg Innov. 2007;14(2):107–12.
7. Cristancho SM, Moussa F, Dubrowski A. A framework-based approach to designing stimulation-augmented surgical education and training programs. Am J Surg. 2011;202:344–51.
8. Kneebone R. Evaluating clinical simulatations for learning procedural skills: a theory-based approach. Acad Med. 2005;80:549–53.
9. Cristancho SM, Hodgson AJ, Pachev G, et al. Assessing cognitive & motor performance in minimally invasive surgery (MAS) for training & tool design. Stud Health Technol Inform. 2006;119:108–13.
10. Aggarwal R, Crantcharow TP, Darzi A. The formula for a successful laparoscopic skills curriculum. J Am Coll Surg. 2007;204:697–705.
11. Stefanidis and Henifrod 2009. Arch Surg. 2009;144(1):77–82.
12. Stefanidis D, Korndorffer Jr JR, Heniford BT, et al. Limited feedback and video tutorials optimize learning and resource utilization during laparoscopic simulator training. Surgery. 2007;142(2):202–6.
13. Fried GM. Lessons from the surgical experience with simulators: incorporation into training and utilization in determining competency. Gastrointest Endosc Clin N Am. 2006;16(3):425–34.
14. Kern DE, Thomas PA, Howard DM, et al. Curriculum development for medical education: a six-step approach. Baltimore: The John Hopkins University Press; 1998.
15. Curriculum planning and development. In: Dent J, Hardan RM. A practical guide for medical teachers. Elsevier Health Sciences, UK, 2009.
16. Ericsson KA. Deliberate practice and the acquisition of maintenance of expert performance in medicine and related domains. Acad Med. 2004;79(10 suppl):S70–81.
17. Ericsson KA, Lehmann AC. Expert and exceptional performance: evidence of maximal adaptation to task constraints. Annu Rev Psychol. 1996;47:273–305.
18. Stefanidis D, Akker CE, Greeny FL. Performance goals on simulators boost resident's demotivation and skills laboratory attendance. J Surg Educ. 2010;67(2):66–70.
19. Magil RA. Motor learning and control. Concepts and application. 7th ed. New York: McGraw-Hill; 2004.
20. van der Meijden OA, Schijven MP. The value of haptic feedback in conventional and robot-assisted minimal invasive surgery and virtual reality training: a current review. Surg Endosc. 2009;23(6):1180–90.
21. Porte MC, Xeroulis G, Reznick RK, et al. Verbal feedback from an expert is more effective than self-accessed feedback about motion, efficiency in learning new surgical skills. Am J Surg. 2007;193(1):105–10.
22. Kruglikova L, Grantcharov TP, Drewes AM, et al. The impact of constructive feedback on training in gastrointestinal endoscopy using high fidelity virtual reality simulation. A randomised controlled trial. Gut. 2010;59(2):181–5.
23. Winstein CJ, Schmidt RA. Reduced frequency of knowledge of results enhances motor skill learning. J Exp Psychol Learn Mem Cogn. 1990;16:677–91.
24. Strandbygaard J. et al. Instructor feedback versus no instructor feedback on performance in a laparoscopic virtual reality simulator: a randomized trial. Ann Surg. 257(5):293 no date.
25. Jowett N, LeBlanc V, Xeroulis G, et al. Surgical skill acquisition with self-directed practice using computer-based video training. Am J Surg. 2007;193(2):237–42.

26. Summers AN, Rinehart GC, Simpson D, et al. Acquisition of surgical skills: a randomised trial of didactic, video tape, and computer-based training. Surgery. 1999;126(2):330–6.
27. Stefanidis D. Optimal Acquisition and assessment of proficiency on simulators in surgery. Surg Clin North Am. 2010;90:475–89.
28. Moulton CA, Dubrowski A, Macrae H, et al. Teaching surgical skills: what kind of practice makes perfect?: a randomized, controlled trial. Ann Surg. 2006;244(3):400–9.
29. Mackay S, Morgan P, Datta V, et al. Practice distribution in procedural skills training: a randomized contolled trial. Surg Endosc. 2002;16(6):957–61.
30. Karni A, Meyer G, Rey-Hipolito C, et al. The acquisition of skilled motor performance: fast and slow experience-driven changes in primary motor cortex. Proc Natl Acad Sci U S A. 1998;95(3):861–8.
31. Walter KC, Acker CE, Heniford BT, et al. Performance goals on simulators boost resident motivation and skills lab attendance. J Am Col Surg. 2008;207(3):S88.
32. Gallagher AG, Ritter EM, Champion H, et al. Virtual reality simulation for the operating room: proficiency-based training as a paradigm shift in surgical skills training. Ann Surg. 2005; 241(2):364–72.
33. Stafanidis D, Heniford BT. The formula for successful laparoscopic skills curriculum. Arch Surg. 2009;144(1):77–82.
34. Madan AK, Harper JL, Taddeucci RJ, et al. Goal-directed laparoscopic training leads to better laparoscopic skills acquisition. Surgery. 2008;144(2):345–50.
35. Brydges R, Carnahan H, Safir O, et al. How effective is self-guided learning of clinical technical skills? It's all about process. Med Educ. 2009;43(6):507–15.
36. Brinkman W, Buzink SN, Alevizos L, de Hingh IH, Jakimowicz JJ. Criterion based laparoscopic training reduces total training time. Surg Endosc. 2012;16(4):1095–101.
37. Issenberg SB, McGaghie WC, Petrusa ER, et al. Features and use of high-fidelity medical simulations that lead to effective learning: a BEME systematic review. Med Teach. 2005;27(1): 10–28.
38. Ali MR, Mowery Y, Kaplan B, et al. Training the novice n laparoscopy. More chalenge is better. Surg Endosc. 2002;16(12):1732–6.
39. Wulf G, Lee TD. Contextual Interference in movements of the same class: differential effects on program and parameter learning. J Mot Behav. 1993;25(4):254–63.
40. Kurahashi A, Leming K, Carnahan H, et al. Effects of expertise, practice and contextual interference on adaptations to visuo-motor MAS alignment. Stud Health Technol Inform. 2008;132:225–9.
41. Stefanidis D, Scerbo MW, Korndorffer Jr JR, et al. Redefining simulator proficiency using automaticity theory. Am J Surg. 2007;193(4):502–6.
42. Pluyter JR, Rutkowski AF, Jakimowicz JJ. Immersive training: breaking the bubble and measuring the heat. Surg Endosc. 2014;28:1545–54.
43. Pluyter JR, Buzink SN, Rutkowski AF, Jakimowicz JJ. Do absorption and realistic distraction influence performance of component task surgerical procedure? Surg Endosc. 2010;24(4): 902–7.
44. Xiao DJ1, Jakimowicz JJ, Albayrak A, Goossens RH. Ergonomic factors on task performance in laparoscopic surgery training. Appl Ergon. 2012;43(3):548–53. doi: 10.1016/j.apergo.2011.08.010.
45. Gallagher AG, Ritter EM, Satava RM. Fundamental principles of validation, and reliability: rigorous science for the assessment of surgical education and training. Surg Endosc. 2003;17(10):1525–9. Epub 2003 Sep 19.
46. Stefanidis D, Korndorffer Jr JR, Markley S, et al. Closing the gap in operative performance between novices and experts: does harder mean better for laparoscopic simulator training. J Am Coll Surg. 2007;205(2):307–13.
47. Kogan JR, Holmboe ES, Hauer KE. Tools for direct observation and assessment of clinical skills of medical trainees: a systematic review. JAMA. 2009;302:1316–26.
48. Ahmed K, Miskovic A, Skovuc D, Darzi A, et al. Observational tools for assessment of procedural skills: a systemic review. Am J Surg. 2011;202:469–80.
49. Epstein RM. Assessment in medical education. N Engl J Med. 2007;356:387–96.

50. Leong JJ, Leff DR, Das A, et al. Validation of orthopaedic bench models for trauma surgery. J Bone Joint Surg Br. 2008;90:958–65.
51. Joice P, Hanna GB, Cuschieri A. Errors enacted during endoscopic surgery – a human reliability analysis. Appl Ergon. 1998;29:409–14.
52. Tang B, Hanna GB, Joice P, et al. Identification and categorization of technical errors by Observational Clinical Human Reliability Assessment (OCHRA) during laparoscopic cholecystectomy. Arch Surg. 2004;139:1215–20.
53. Tang B, Hanna GB, Cuschieri A. Analysis of errors enacted by surgical trainees during skills training courses. Surgery. 2005;138:14–20.
54. Tang B, Hanna GB, Carter F, et al. Competence assessment of laparoscopic operative and cognitive skills: Objective Structured Clinical Examination (OSCE) or Observational Clinical Human Reliability Assessment (OCHRA). World J Surg. 2006;30:527–34.
55. Vassiliou MC, Kaneva PA, Poulose BK, Dunkin BJ, Marks JM, Sadik R, Sroka G, Anvari M, Thaler K, Adrales GL, Hazey JW, Lightdale JR, Velanovich V, Swanstrom LL, Mellinger JD, Fried GM. Global Assessment of Gastrointestinal Endoscopic Skills (GAGES): a valid measurement tool for technical skills in flexible endoscopy. Surg Endosc. 2010;24(8):1834–41. doi:10.1007/s00464-010-0882-8. Epub 2010 Jan 29.
56. Ottowa. Performance in assessment : consensus statement and recommandations. From: http://www.academia.edu/2550139/Performance_in_assessment_Consensus_statement_and_recommendations_from_the_Ottawa_conference.
57. Miskovic D, Wyles SM, Francis NK, Rockall TA, Kennedy RH, Hanna GB on behalf of the National Training Programme in Laparoscopic Colorectal Surgery. Laparoscopic Colorectal Competency Assessment Tool (LCAT) for the National Training Programme in England. Ann Surg. 2013;257(3):476–82.
58. Padney VA, Wolfe JH, Black SA, et al. Self-assessment of technical skill in surgery: the need for expert feedback. Ann R Coll Surg Engl. 2008;90(4):286–90.
59. MacDonald J, Williams RG, Rogers DA. Self-assessment in simulation-based surgical skills training. Am J Surg. 2003;185:319–22.
60. Falchikov NB, Boud D. Student self-assessment in higher education: a meta-analysis. Rev Educ Res. 1989;59:395–430.
61. Brewster LP, Risucci DA, Joehl RJ, et al. Comparison of resident self-assessment with trained faculty and standardized patient assessment of clinical and technical skills in a structured educational module. Am J Surg. 2008;195:1–4.
62. Arora S, Miskovic D, Hull L, et al. Self vs expert assessment of technical and non-technical skills in high fidelity simulation. Am J Surg. 2011;202:500–6.
63. Moorthy K, Munz Y, Adams S, et al. Self-assessment of performance among surgical trainees during simulated operating theater. Am J Surg. 2006;192:114–8.
64. McKimm J. Curriculum design and development. From: www.faculty.londondeanery.ac.uk/…/Curriculum_de looks to be incomplete
65. Dunn WR, Hamilton DD, Harden RM. Techniques of identifying competencies needed by doctors. Med Teach. 1985;7(1):15–25.
66. Jakimowicz JJ, Cuschieri A. Time for evidence-based minimal access surgery training – simulate or sink. Surg Endosc. 2005;19:1–3.
67. Jakimowicz JJ, Fingerhut A. Simulation in surgery. Br J Surg. 2009;96:563–4.
68. Hasson HM. Core competency in laparoendoscopic surgery. JSLS. 2006;10:16–20.
69. Schijven MP. Virtual reality simulation for laparoscopic cholecystectomy – the process of validation and implementation in the surgical curriculum outlined. Phd thesis, University of Leiden, Leiden; 2005.
70. Buzink SN, Schiappa JM, Bicha Castelo H, Fingerhut A, Hanna G, Jakimowicz JJ. The laparoscopic surgical skills A, programme: setting the European standard. Revista portuguesa de cirurgia. 2012;20:33–40.
71. Buzink SN, Soltes M, Fingerhut A, Hanna G, Jakimowicz JJ. The laparoscopic surgical skills programme: setting the European standard. Videosurg Mininv. 2012;7:188–92.

Chapter 3
Simulation and Training in Minimal Access Surgery

Alexander Harris, Fernando Bello, and Roger Kneebone

Introduction

The aim of this chapter is to provide readers of all backgrounds with a general introduction to simulation and training in minimal access surgery. The chapter will encompass: the relevance of simulation training to modern surgical practice; the arguments for and against each of the various modalities described; and potential emergent directions and technologies.

Definitions

In this first section, the key terms that are relevant to the field of surgical simulation have been defined for the reader as they will be used in the context of this chapter. However, it should be noted that these definitions are heterogeneous across the simulation literature such that interpretations in other texts may differ from those presented here.

Simulation and Simulators

Describing the distinction between simulation and a simulator is a commonly encountered difficulty. This chapter defines simulation as a technique, and a simulator as a technology [1]. *Simulation* is therefore utilised as an umbrella term

A. Harris, MBBS, MRCS (Eng) (✉) • F. Bello, PhD • R. Kneebone, PhD, FRCS
Centre for Engagement and Simulation Science, Imperial College London, 3rd Floor Chelsea and Westminster Hospital (Academic Surgery), 369 Fulham Road, London SW10 9NH, UK
e-mail: alexander.harris00@imperial.ac.uk; f.bello@imperial.ac.uk; r.kneebone@imperial.ac.uk

N. Francis et al. (eds.), *Training in Minimal Access Surgery*,
DOI 10.1007/978-1-4471-6494-4_3

for "artificial alternatives to clinical practice" [2] that recreate educationally rich scenarios within a learner-centred context, whereas a *simulator* is the training modality or device used within a simulation.

Fidelity, Validity and Reliability

Fidelity describes how faithfully a simulation or simulator represents real-life circumstances, such that, for all intents and purposes, it is a marker of *realism* [3]. The more *immersive* a simulation, the greater the realism, as the participant is able to suspend their disbelief of the artificial nature of the scenario. A common misconception is that cost and fidelity are directly proportional, or that high fidelity is better than low fidelity. In fact, the required fidelity for a simulation should be judged solely against its aims, and its cost-effectiveness against its objectively measurable impact.

Validity is the degree to which a test measures what it purports to measure. There are several different types: *face validity* is the degree to which a test represents reality; *content validity* is the degree to which the domain being measured is actually measured; *construct validity* is the degree to which the test measures the construct it is designed to measure or can distinguish between different levels of performance; *concurrent validity* compares the new test against the current gold standard; and *predictive validity* is the degree to which the test can predict expected or future performance [4, 5].

Reliability is a measure of the consistency and reproducibility of results, quantified on a scale between 0 and 1, where 1 equates to absolute agreement. In the published literature, a score of 0.8 and above is usually deemed acceptable. If a test is performed twice on an individual, without learning, the result is expected to be identical. This is known as *test-retest reliability. Inter-rater reliability* measures the agreement between independent observers of the same test [5].

Relevance of Simulation to Modern Surgical Practice

The latter part of the twentieth century heralded a watershed in operative surgical practice, with minimal access techniques replacing open surgery as the gold standard for many common procedures performed across a range of specialties. However, this presented the surgical community with a significant challenge, as fully trained open surgeons were required to adapt to the technical demands of a minimal access approach without compromising patient safety or outcomes.

With the subsequent climate of change impacting upon surgical education and practice worldwide [6–9], simulation – traditionally associated with the military and aviation industry – has been proposed as a potential adjunct to clinical experience at all levels of training [10–17].

A recent review critiqued forty years of simulation research and identified twelve key features and best practices of simulation based medical education [18]. This review presented evidence in support of: feedback; deliberate practice; curriculum integration; outcome measurement; simulation fidelity; skill acquisition and maintenance; mastery learning; transfer to practice; team training; high-stakes testing; instructor training; and educational and professional context.

Nonetheless, uptake of simulation training has been hindered by scepticism relating to its accessibility, limitations, translational benefits, cost-effectiveness, and research study designs [19]. Therefore, in order to become established in mainstream practice, a stronger research evidence-base and a cultural shift in attitude towards simulation are required.

Simulation Training

Since the early 1990s, there has been a dramatic rise in the number of minimal access surgical simulators that are commercially available. Due to various constraints, these simulators simplify the complex nature of surgery down to task-based procedures. The published literature is therefore heavily weighted toward the objective evaluation of these task-based simulators rather than descriptions of innovative approaches to simulation, which tend not to be seen as research. As such, the available literature provides an incomplete representation of the current and actual state of the art [20]. In the next section, the commonest types of surgical simulators are identified and the current evidence for and against their use is discussed.

Virtual Reality

Pioneered by the computer scientist Jaron Lanier, virtual reality "refers to a computer-generated representation of an environment that allows sensory interaction, thus giving the impression of actually being present" [21]. First generation virtual reality simulators focused upon developing trainees' basic minimal access skills e.g., manipulating objects in three dimensions. As computer graphics evolved and improved, second generation simulators were able to place these skills in surgical context. Third generation simulators went a step further in recreating multiple stages of entire surgical procedures, whilst also moving beyond psychomotor skills to incorporate cognitive training in the steps of a procedure and the relevant anatomy. Current, fourth generation, simulators now provide a holistic approach that combines diagnostic tutorials and indications for surgery, with traditional procedural tasks [22]. Indeed, a recent Cochrane review concluded that "virtual reality training improves standard surgical training" [23].

MIST-VR® (Mentice, Gothenburg, Sweden) is one of the earliest, validated, minimal access virtual reality simulators. It was designed for training basic psychomotor skills where trainees could complete standardised tasks, such as grasping and manipulating objects, and receive immediate feedback on objective measures of their technical performance e.g., the total number of errors made and path length (distance travelled) for each hand. This data could then be saved and used to compare an individual's performance longitudinally, in order to demonstrate skill acquisition, or cross-sectionally for comparison amongst peer group performance [24]. It has been proven that these psychomotor skills are transferrable to the operating theatre, with trainees demonstrating significantly shorter duration of dissection and fewer errors during laparoscopic cholecystectomy [25].

LapSim® (Surgical Science, Gothenburg, Sweden) advanced the field by providing modules covering basic psychomotor skills, tasks, and operations with improved realism through deformable on-screen graphics. However, the original LapSim®, like MIST-VR®, lacked haptic (touch or force) feedback. Nonetheless, validation studies have shown that virtual reality training using LapSim® moves the trainees' skill acquisition out of theatre through psychomotor skills transfer from simulation to the clinical domain [26]. There is also evidence to suggest that surgical performance is improved when LapSim® is used as a pre-operative surgical warm-up [27].

LapMentor™ (Simbionix, Cleveland, OH) added haptic feedback to a range of basic and advanced minimal access procedures [28]. However, a significant benefit from the addition of haptic feedback to trainees' skill acquisition is yet to be demonstrated [29], although it is suspected to improve performance in advanced tasks and procedures [30].

There are several recognised practical concerns regarding virtual reality simulators [31]. Cost is the most significant as, in addition to the purchase price, there are also storage and maintenance costs to consider. In particular, the fact that technology is evolving and advancing so rapidly means that organisations want cheap, easy to install, software upgrades to be made available. Furthermore, cost-effectiveness dictates that the departments implementing such technology must perceive the benefit of trainees using these simulators positively offset against their financial outgoings. Whilst there is evidence to support faster operating times and fewer errors, there is no published evidence currently describing a financial saving.

Fundamentally, not enough is known about maximising laparoscopic skills acquisition in virtual reality. This, in turn, provides critics with the legitimacy to question, somewhat rhetorically, why trainees are encouraged to spend their time in a virtual environment when they are struggling to receive adequate clinical experience.

Synthetic Physical Models

Synthetic physical models have traditionally been used for teaching and assessing basic clinical skills across a range of undergraduate and postgraduate grades. Over time, these models have progressed to provide anatomically accurate training tools for a range of surgical procedures across a variety of surgical specialties, including minimal access surgery.

Despite a lack of research papers systematically validating their use [32], specially designed programmes often incorporate these relatively low-cost, low-fidelity, models in laparoscopic video (box) trainers for the targeted training of junior surgeons. At this level, the emphasis is placed on learning the cognitive steps of an operative procedure, and practicing the fundamental, often counter-intuitive, psychomotor skills involved.

Whilst the materials used are predominantly single use, limited in terms of their tissue handling properties, and generally unable to support the use of diathermy, they are also cheap, readily available, and allow trainees to gain confidence and competence in a procedure within a learner-centred laboratory setting.

Animal Models

Despite live animal operating being prohibited in the UK, (but not overseas), organs harvested from animals that are slaughtered for human consumption are permitted to be used for surgical training. However, both suppliers and end-users are closely regulated and so such training is generally restricted to specialist regional centres that may be less accessible to trainees.

Despite these practical considerations, there are several benefits to simulations involving ex-vivo animal tissue. Firstly, the purchase price per unit is markedly cheaper than other modalities. Secondly, despite structural anatomical differences, the tissue texture is closer to human than virtual reality or synthetic physical models. Thirdly, diathermy can be used. As such ex-vivo animal tissue is often preferred for simulations involving advanced surgical trainees although, as with synthetic physical models, there is a lack of evidence-based research systematically evaluating their use [32].

Human Cadavers

Human cadavers are a scarce resource in the UK as people rarely donate their body to medical science. However, the UK Human Tissue Act has recently changed to permit the use of human cadavers for learning procedures – a move that aligns UK policy with existing overseas practise – providing that the donor has been appropriately consented pre-mortem.

Whilst undergraduate cadaveric dissection is increasingly being phased out, more senior trainees and consultants are attracted to simulation courses offering human cadaveric dissection due to its advantages with respect to anatomy, surgical authenticity, and realism – in particular with fresh frozen cadavers [33].

It is possible to perform a range of contextualised procedures with each cadaver, across a range of specialties, in order to maximise its cost-effectiveness. However, it is imperative to sequence the procedures according to the anatomy that will be disturbed or preserved following each completed task [34]. If performed successfully, new procedures, techniques, and technologies can be learned in a safe environment that is the closest available to live human operating.

Despite such benefits, human cadaveric simulation is expensive. This is due in part to the limited availability of cadavers in the UK, as well as the cost of facilities that are suitably equipped and licensed to handle them. As such, this simulation modality is generally only available in regional training centres.

The Importance of Context

The commonest approach to minimal access surgical skills teaching is task-based simulation, where the focus is placed upon developing technical skills e.g., laparoscopic suturing. Whilst deliberate practice of a new, or weak, skill has demonstrable benefits [35], one limitation of simulation is how skills are generally taught in isolation. This is highly unrealistic when considering the clinical environment, where a surgeon is frequently required to demonstrate a range of skills both simultaneously and interchangeably. Indeed, it has been postulated that context aids the development of such expertise [36]. Our research group at Imperial College London has pioneered the concepts of physical and temporal context in simulation training and researched the added benefits that they can provide.

Physical Context

The physical context of a simulation relates to environmental factors, such as the setting, choice of simulator, and the nature of surgery. As surgery is heavily sense-based, surgical simulations must attempt to recreate the sights, sounds, smells, and touch of the operating theatre, in order to be most effective. Such physical contextualisation provides an appropriate backdrop to the simulation and aids participant immersion within the scenario (Fig. 3.1).

In situ simulation (performed in the actual clinical setting) is still in its infancy, but has demonstrated potential for use in multidisciplinary team training e.g., trauma and cardiopulmonary resuscitation scenarios [37]. However, in situ simulation for surgery is limited by the accessibility of the operating theatre with respect to cost and clinical demand. Many teaching hospitals have therefore established static simulation facilities with dedicated staff, but these can also prove costly, difficult for trainees to access, and are subsequently often under-used. More recently, portable and mobile simulation facilities have been designed to counter such issues [38]. These modalities specifically target trainees who would otherwise struggle to

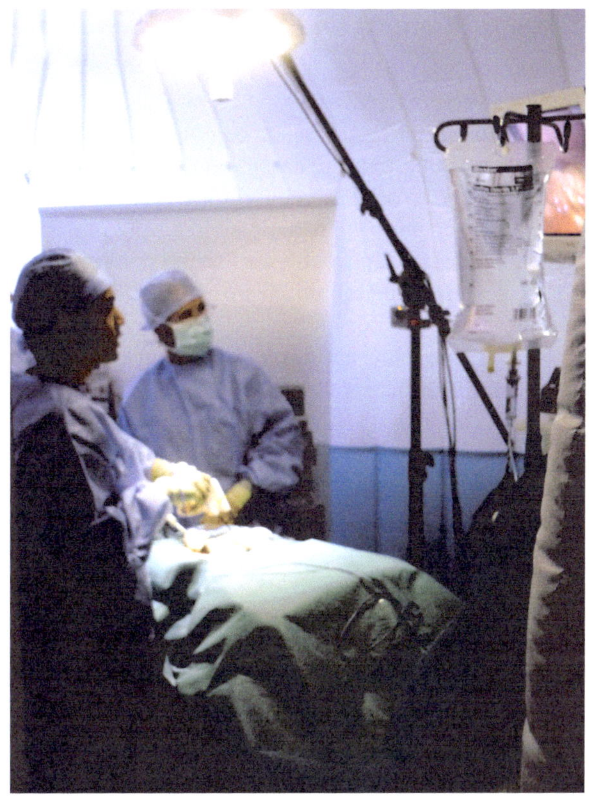

Fig. 3.1 Physically contextualised minimal access surgical simulation training using a video (box) trainer and ex vivo porcine tissue

routinely access specialist centres, with evidence to suggest that the facilities and participant experiences are comparable to their more illustrious, and expensive, counterparts [39–41].

We have previously considered the various simulation modalities available for minimal access surgery training. However, it is also of vital importance for training that surgeons are able to perform simulated procedures in the manner, and with the tools, that they would use in real life.

Physical contextualisation can therefore range from the simple towel draping of a virtual reality surgical simulator, to hybrid models that enable actual surgery to be performed by providing local context of the operative field. Examples include using a synthetic silicone skin over the outer casing of a video (box) trainer, coupled with an internal anatomical model that permits modular substitution of anatomy with e.g., porcine tissue, such as the liver and gallbladder or a section of small bowel. This flexibility permits more authentic surgical simulation through the facilitation of modern surgical practices and procedures.

However, physical contextualisation can be resource and faculty intensive. By incorporating roles for anaesthetic and scrub staff, who add authenticity to the simulation by recreating the social aspect of surgery, the educational value of the exercise and participant immersion are increased whilst the financial costs per group may be reduced.

Temporal Context and Sequential Simulation

Temporal context relates to time. Whilst a patient's surgical journey may take weeks, months, or even years to complete, simulation offers an opportunity to distil this sequence of events in a process called "sequential simulation" [42]. For instance, a trainee may be asked to consent a simulated patient (medically trained actor or actress) pre-operatively, participate in a fully immersive operative team simulation for that procedure, and then examine the same simulated patient post-operatively.

The benefits of this approach are two-fold. Firstly, by contextualising the operation in time, place, and person, trainee engagement is increased. Secondly, concomitant factors e.g., communication skills can be taught and/ or tested. Such a holistic approach transcends the technical task, testing the trainees' understanding and explanation of a procedure, through effective communication of its indications, risks, and benefits to a patient. Faculty have the opportunity to standardise operative scenarios across training grades, or tailor them according to trainee performance – pushing stronger candidates and supporting weaker ones. Post-operatively, a prosthetic and make-up artist is able to deliver authentic surgical wounds, such that trainees' ability to identify and manage potential complications is addressed, where appropriate (Fig. 3.2).

Whilst such simulations may appear financially and logistically demanding to implement routinely, the results of pilot studies performed at Imperial College London in association with the London Deanery support plans for wider trainee access to this form of training modality.

Surgical Simulation – the Future

There are a number of exciting new developments that may impact upon the future of simulation training for minimal access surgery. These developments have been driven by working time restrictions reducing the exposure of surgical trainees to clinical and operative episodes, an increased emphasis on improving patient safety and the rapid evolution of technology. Six of the most practical and innovative ideas are discussed here.

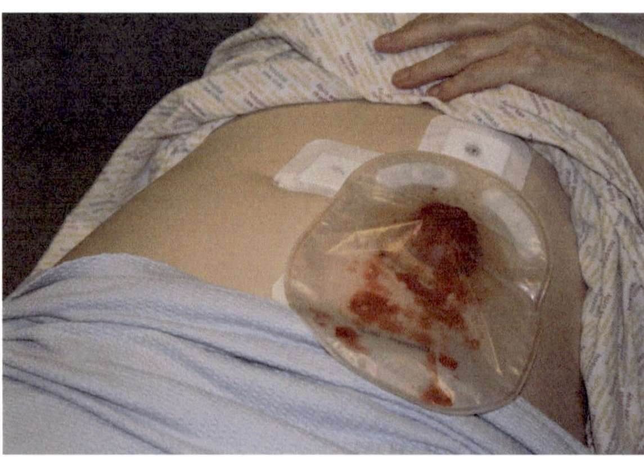

Fig. 3.2 A simulated patient's post-operative abdomen with a (silicone) end colostomy

Specialist Simulation Training Centres

Given the current climate affecting surgical education, and high level support in favour of simulation training, there is a growing trend towards establishing specialist simulation centres [43]. These centres offer trainees the facilities to consolidate and supplement their clinical experience, often through co-ordinated and structured regional training programmes. Other centres provide trainees with unrestricted access and the opportunity for self-directed learning. At present, there is no clear evidence in favour of one approach over the other [44, 45].

Increasingly, trainees are purchasing, or being provided with, their own personal minimal access training devices. This negates the need, and cost, of a specialised centre whilst permitting the trainee to practice at their own convenience. However, in the absence of feedback from a trainer, there is a risk of uncorrected mistakes and poor technique becoming habitual.

Simulation Curriculum

The development of a comprehensive, valid and reliable, simulation curriculum for surgical training is not a new concept. Whilst excellent basic skills courses exist e.g., Fundamentals of Laparoscopic Surgery program [46], and significant efforts towards developing procedure specific curricula have been made [47], as yet, no definitive simulation curriculum for advanced minimal access surgical skills training exists. The current state of the art relates to specific tasks, performed on specific simulators, even though there is little cross comparison between simulators or evidence correlating simulation competence with clinical competence across a range of procedures. It has therefore been proposed that curriculum development should be embraced as an iterative process that requires concurrent validation [48].

The London Deanery general surgery training programme is unique in following an integrated simulation curriculum extending over the entire duration of surgical training. It is taught by specialist trainers, trainee attendance and performance is monitored throughout, individualised feedback is provided, and trainees' progress is recorded through regular appraisals. However, at present, only feasibility and participant acceptability have been established [49].

Competence for Clinical Practice

Whilst simulation is championed as an adjunct to, rather than a substitute for, clinical experience, a controversial yet potential next step is for surgical trainees to be required to demonstrate competence in simulation prior to being permitted to perform clinical procedures on patients. This transition makes sense from an ethical and patient safety perspective, with regard to moving the trainees' skill acquisition out of theatre and maximising the value of subsequent clinical episodes. However, it would be difficult to enforce given existing workplace pressures.

Procedure Rehearsal

First described in 2001, patient specific virtual reality procedural rehearsal is a potentially revolutionary emergent technology. The technique involves surgeons using patient scans for pre-operative procedural planning tailored to the individual patient's anatomy and pathology. It facilitates cognitive and psychomotor rehearsal, and improves the prospects of success for complex procedures by easing the burden of intra-operative decision-making and allowing surgeons to select the most appropriate surgical approach in advance of the operation, thereby optimising patient safety and achievable patient outcomes [50].

Testing and Integration of New Technologies

Technological advancements have been a key driver for innovation in minimal access surgery, but safely translating promising research to the operating theatre is a major issue. Simulation offers one viable solution for trialling new technology in a realistic clinical environment. Scientists are afforded the opportunity to iron-out previously unforeseen potential difficulties, whilst end-users can learn to use the technology under supervision, ask questions, and voice concerns away from the pressures of the clinical workplace and without risk to patient safety. Indeed patients and the lay public may be invited, and even encouraged, to join in this process [51]. This approach has been successfully piloted at Imperial College London and opens up potential new avenues for how clinical trials may be run in the future.

Tuition and Maintenance of Open Surgical Skills

As a generation of surgeons are predominantly trained in minimal access approaches to surgery, an interesting development has been the loss of traditional open surgical skills. However, the potential requirement for conversion to an open approach remains and dictates that open surgical skills must still be taught and maintained. Simulation is the ideal environment for practicing rare and once-in-a-lifetime scenarios, often with tuition from trainers who performed such procedures when they were commonplace e.g., open cholecystectomy. Consequently, the requirements of surgical simulation training are expected to come full circle [52].

Chapter Summary

Minimal access surgery is a rapidly evolving field. As such, it is imperative that surgical education and training responds in an innovative and timely manner, for present surgical trainees to be adequately and appropriately prepared for the demands of their nascent careers. Simulation offers one potential solution.

This chapter has adopted a broad perspective in considering the role that simulation has to play in minimal access surgery training. It has explored its relevance to modern surgical practice, identified evidence for the strengths and weaknesses of existing training modalities, and discussed several of its conceivable future directions.

References

1. Gaba D. The future vision of simulation in health care. Qual Safe Health Care. 2004; 13:i2–10.
2. Kneebone R. Simulation in surgical training: educational issues and practical implications. Med Educ. 2003;37:267–77.
3. Brydges R, Carnahan H, Rose D, Rose L, Dubrowski A. Coordinating progressive levels of simulation fidelity to maximise educational benefit. Acad Med. 2010;85:806–12.
4. Moorthy K, Munz Y, Sarker S, Darzi A. Objective assessment of technical skills in surgery. Br Med J. 2003;327:1032–7.
5. Ratanawongsa N, Thomas P, Marinopoulos S, Dorman T, Wilson L, Ashar B, et al. The reported validity and reliability of methods for evaluating continuing medical education: a systematic review. Acad Med. 2008;83:274–83.
6. Directive 2003/88/EC of the European Parliament and of the Council of 4 November 2003 concerning certain aspects of the organisation of working time. Official Journal L 299, 18/11/2003 P. 0009–0019.
7. Tooke J. Final report of the independent inquiry into Modernising Medical Careers. MMC Inquiry. London: Aldridge Press. 2007. See http://www.mmcinquiry.org.uk/draft.htm.
8. Chikwe J, de Souza A, Pepper J. No time to train the surgeons. Br Med J. 2004;328:418–9.
9. Grantcharov T, Reznick R. Training tomorrow's surgeons: what are we looking for and how can we achieve it? ANZ J Surg. 2009;79:104–7.
10. Donaldson L. 150 years of the Annual Report of the Chief Medical Officer. 2008 [10 Aug 2013]; Available from: webarchive.nationalarchives.gov.uk/+/http://www.dh.gov.uk/en/publicationsandstatistics/publications/annualreports/dh_096206.
11. Temple J. Time for Training. A review of the impact of the European Working Time Directive on the quality of training. 2010 [10 Aug 2013]; Available from: http://www.mee.nhs.uk/PDF/14274 Bookmark Web Version.pdf.
12. Aggarwal R, Darzi A. From scalpel to simulator: a surgical journey. Surgery. 2009;145:1–4.
13. Choy I, Okrainec A. Simulation in surgery: perfecting the practice. Surg Clin North Am. 2010;90:457–73.
14. Jakimowicz J, Cuschieri A. Time for evidence-based minimal access surgery training: simulate or sink. Surg Endosc. 2005;19:1521–2.
15. Satava R. Surgical education and surgical simulation. World J Surg. 2001;25:1484–9.
16. Sturm L, Windsor J, Cosman P, Cregan P, Hewett P, Maddern G. A systematic review of skills transfer after surgical simulation training. Ann Surg. 2008;248:166–79.

17. Windsor J. Role of simulation in surgical education and training. ANZ J Surg. 2009;79: 127–32.
18. McGaghie W, Issenberg S, Petrusa E, Scalese R. A critical review of simulation-based medical education research: 2003–2009. Med Educ. 2010;44:50–63.
19. Sutherland L, Middleton P, Anthony A, Hamdorf J, Cregan P, Scott D, et al. Surgical simulation: a systematic review. Ann Surg. 2006;243:291–300.
20. Regehr G. Trends in medical education research. Acad Med. 2004;79:939–47.
21. Coleman J, Nduka C, Darzi A. Virtual reality and laparoscopic surgery. Br J Surg. 1994;81: 1709–11.
22. Undre S, Darzi A. Laparoscopy simulators. J Endourol. 2007;21:274–9.
23. Gurusamy K, Aggarwal R, Palanivelu L, Davidson B. Virtual reality training for surgical trainees in laparoscopic surgery. Cochrane Database Syst Rev. 2009;(1):CD006575.
24. Wilson M, Middlebrook A, Sutton C, Stone R, McCloy RMISTVR. A virtual reality trainer for laparoscopic surgery assesses performance. Ann R Coll Surg Engl. 1997;79:403–4.
25. Seymour N, Gallagher A, Roman S, O'Brien M, Bansal V, Andersen D, et al. Virtual reality training improves operating room performance. Ann Surg. 2002;236:458–64.
26. Larsen C, Soerensen J, Grantcharov T, Dalsgaard T, Schouenborg L, Ottosen C, et al. Effect of virtual reality training on laparoscopic surgery: randomised controlled trial. Br Med J. 2009; 338:b1802.
27. Catalyud D, Arora S, Aggarwal R, Kruglikova I, Schulze S, Funch-Jensen P, et al. Warm-up in a virtual reality environment improves performance in the operating room. Ann Surg. 2010;251:1181–5.
28. Andreatta P, Woodrum D, Birkmeyer J, Yellamanchilli R, Doherty G, Gauger P, et al. Laparoscopic skills are improved with LapMentor Training: results of a randomized, double-blinded study. Ann Surg. 2006;243:854–60.
29. Thompson J, Leonard A, Doarn C, Roesch M, Broderick T. Limited value of haptics in virtual reality laparoscopic cholecystectomy training. Surg Endosc. 2011;25:1107–14.
30. Panait L, Akkary E, Bell R, Roberts K, Dudrick S, Duffy A. The role of haptic feedback in laparoscopic simulation training. J Surg Res. 2009;156:312–6.
31. Bashir G. Technology and medicine: the evolution of virtual reality simulation in laparoscopic training. Med Teach. 2010;32:558–61.
32. Aucar J, Groch N, Troxel S, Eubanks S. A review of surgical simulation with attention to validation methodology. Surg Laparosc Endosc Percutan Tech. 2005;15:82–9.
33. Wyles S, Miskovic D, Ni Z, Acheson A, Maxwell-Armstrong C, Longman R, et al. Analysis of laboratory-based laparoscopic colorectal surgery workshops within the English National Training Programme. Surg Endosc. 2011;25:1559–66.
34. Harris A. Distributed simulation and soft preserve cadavers in surgical simulation. Granada: SESAM; 2011.
35. Ericsson K, Charness N, Feltovich P, Hoffman R, editors. The Cambridge handbook of expertise and expert performance. New York: Cambridge University Press; 2006.
36. Mylopoulos M, Regehr G. Putting the expert together again. Med Educ. 2011;45:920–6.
37. Rosen M, Hunt E, Pronovost P, Federowicz M, Weaver S. In situ simulation in continuing education for health care professions: a systematic review. J Contin Educ Health Prof. 2012;32:243–54.
38. Kneebone R, Arora S, King D, Bello F, Sevdalis N, Kassab E, et al. Distributed simulation – accessible immersive training. Med Teach. 2010;32:65–70.
39. Kassab E, Tun J, Arora S, King D, Ahmed K, Miskovic D, et al. "Blowing up the barriers" in surgical training: exploring and validating the concept of distributed simulation. Ann Surg. 2011;254:1059–65.
40. Kassab E, Kyaw Tun J, Kneebone R. A novel approach to contextualized surgical simulation training. Simul Healthc. 2012;7:155–61.
41. Harris A, Kassab E, Tun JK, Kneebone R. Distributed Simulation in surgical training: an off-site feasibility study. Med Teach. 2013;35(4):e1078–81.
42. Kneebone R. Simulation, safety and surgery. Qual Safe Health Care. 2010;19:i47–52.

43. Sachdeva A, Pellegrini C, Johnson K. Support for simulation-based surgical education through American College of Surgeons – Accredited Education Institutes. World J Surg. 2008;32: 196–207.
44. Chang L, Petros J, Hess D, Rotondi C, Babineau T. Integrating simulation into a surgical residency program: is voluntary participation effective? Surg Endosc. 2007;21:418–21.
45. Snyder C, Vandromme M, Tyra S, Hawn M. Proficiency-based laparoscopic and endoscopic training with virtual reality simulators: a comparison of proctored and independent approaches. J Surg Educ. 2009;66:201–7.
46. Swanstrom L, Fried G, Hoffman K, Soper N. Beta test results of a new system assessing competence in laparoscopic surgery. J Am Coll Surg. 2006;202:62–9.
47. Palter V, Orzech N, Reznick R, Grantcharov T. Validation of a structured training and assessment curriculum for technical skill acquisition in minimally invasive surgery: a randomized controlled trial. Ann Surg. 2013;257:224–30.
48. Sweet R, Hananel D, Lawrenz F. A unified approach to validation, reliability, and education study design for surgical technical skills training. Arch Surg. 2010;145:197–201.
49. Hanna G, Mavroveli S, Marchington S, Allen-Mersh T, Paice E, Standfield N. The feasibility and acceptability of integrating regular centralised laboratory-based skills training into a surgical training programme. Med Teach. 2012;34:e827–32.
50. Willaert W, Aggarwal R, Van Herzeele I, Cheshire N, Vermassen F. Recent advancements in medical simulation: patient-specific virtual reality simulation. World J Surg. 2012;36:1703–12.
51. Explore surgery. [10 Aug 2013]; Available from: http://www.exploresurgery.com.
52. Kneebone R, Woods A. Recapturing the history of surgical practice through simulation-based re-enactment. Med Hist. 2014;58:106–21.

Chapter 4
Teaching Basic Laparoscopic Skills

Parul J. Shukla, Sameer Sharma, and Abe Fingerhut

Introduction

"See one, do one, teach one" is the basic mantra of teaching medical and surgical skills attributed to William Halsted [1]. As clinicians we will all be called to teach and each one will develop their own style through experience. This chapter serves as a guide to the fundamentals to be considered when teaching basic laparoscopic skills to trainees. 'Good' teaching has great power to influence a trainee to develop good surgical 'habits'. Good teaching will pay dividends in the surgical careers of trainees and help them to become good trainers when they attain suitable proficiency.

An effective training program starts with a route to facilitate teaching good habits. Most, if not all, senior surgeons know more than one way of accomplishing a technical manoeuvre, but teaching a standardized approach is important in the first instance. Personal embellishments can be added once the student has acquired those fundamental standardized skills. Later, periodic observation by an expert is helpful

P.J. Shukla, MD, MS, FRCS, FACRSI (✉)
Surgery, Weill Cornell Medical College & New York Presbyterian Hospital,
1161 York Avenue, Apt 11C, New York, NY 10065, USA
e-mail: PAS2026@MED.CORNELL.EDU

S. Sharma, MD
New York Presbyterian Hospital & Weil Cornell Medical College,
New York City, NY 10065, USA
e-mail: sksharma14@gmail.com

A. Fingerhut, MD, DSC (Hon), FACS
Section for Surgical Research (Prof Uranues), Department of Surgery,
Medical University of Graz, Auenbruggerplatz 29,
8036 Graz, Austria

First Department of Surgery (Prof Leandros), University of Athens,
Hippokration University Hospital, Athens, Greece
e-mail: abefingerhut@aol.com

N. Francis et al. (eds.), *Training in Minimal Access Surgery*,
DOI 10.1007/978-1-4471-6494-4_4

to ensure that the learner is progressing and to correct bad habits before they become ingrained.

Once a basic skill is taught, the learner should have an opportunity to practice at his/her own pace with performance measured to provide indications of progress. Most studies show that dispersed learning over an extensive period of time provides a more effective learning method compared to 'cramming'.

Goal Setting

The first step to train a trainee is to set a goal or multiple goals. Trainees enter learning activities with previous experience, personal-goals and an innate self-efficacy for goal attainment. The trainer must judge the trainee's competence, aptitude and willingness to learn. Each goal must have an appropriate time period attached to this. For instance, this may be 'by the end of this operation I want you to be able to insert an umbilical port', to 'by the end of your 4 month placement with me you will be able to perform a complete laparoscopic cholecystectomy with me assisting.' In studies, specific, challenging goals led more often to higher performance than easy goals, 'do your best' goals or no goals [2, 3]. So setting clear goals is a must.

When trainees see satisfactory goal advancement, they feel assured of their improving skills. This in turn leads students to set new challenging goals (in conjunction with the trainer) and progress can be attained [4].

Training Schematic (Fig. 4.1)

The training of basic laparoscopic skills can be divided into inside the operating room (OR) or outside the OR. Both arenas offer unique opportunities for learning and acquiring skills.

As a surgeon's career progresses from a novice trainee to an expert, training will most likely happen in conjunction both outside and inside the OR. Skills gained outside the OR can then be used inside the OR to build their skill level. Throughout the training period, a trainee's progress should be reviewed regularly and goals refined according to his or her needs.

Training Laparoscopic Skills Outside the OR

The rapid expansion of the world-wide-web and speedy dissemination of information has enabled sharing of knowledge in an accessible and intuitive manner. The relative shortening of trainee working hours has also led to an expansion of training opportunities outside the OR. Training literature is available through relevant

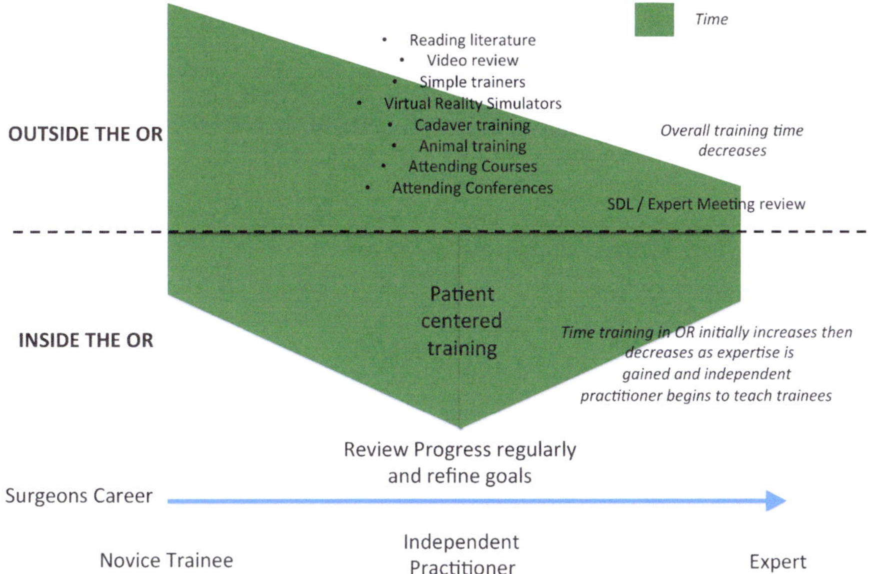

Fig. 4.1 A summary of training evolution during a trainees career to becoming a trainer expert. Green shading denotes time spent both outside and inside the operating room in training activities. As an individual's career progresses the focus and duration of training activities will reflect the needs and responsibilities of that individual

websites and video-upload sites have an ever-increasing number of surgical training videos that can be used by the trainer [5] and trainee. Caution by trainers has to be given to the quality and methods taught in these videos, but this represents an exciting change to training methods in recent times.

Governing Body Accredited Training Programs

Accredited training programs for trainees are available in many countries. These courses follow the curriculum closely and represent an efficient way to attain basic skills outside of the OR [6, 7]. The Fundamentals to Laparoscopic Surgery course (FLS) is one example of this. It is a comprehensive web-based education module that includes a hands-on skills training component and assessment tool designed to teach the physiology, fundamental knowledge, and technical skills required in basic laparoscopic surgery. The goal is to provide surgical residents, fellows and practicing physicians an opportunity to learn the fundamentals of laparoscopic surgery in a consistent, scientifically accepted format; and to test cognitive, surgical decision-making, and technical skills, all with the goal of improving the quality of patient care. The FLS program content has been endorsed by the American College of Surgeons (ACS) and is a joint educational offering of SAGES and ACS [8] (Table 4.1).

Table 4.1 Skills fundamental to laparoscopic surgery (FLS)

Depth perception using monocular optical system
Operating through a trocar (lever effect, decreased degrees of freedom)
Operating with long instruments with dampened force feedback
Use of non-dominant hand
Use of angled laparoscope
Transferring objects between long instruments placed through fixed access points in body wall (trocars)
Precise cutting with both hands using laparoscopic instruments, placed through trocars, using monocular optical system
Use of ligating loops to control hollow tubular structures
Cannulation Suturing and knot tying with intracorporeal and extracorporeal techniques using laparoscopic instruments

Training Ergonomics

The increased technological complexity and sometimes poorly adapted equipment have led to increased complaints of surgeon fatigue and discomfort during laparoscopic surgery. Teaching the trainee to understanding ergonomics cannot only enhance learning but also reduce physical strain and fatigue.

The importance of ergonomics in the setting of laparoscopy cannot be overemphasized. Studies have shown that correct ergonomics can reduce key skill acquisition time [9].

Surgeon's Position

A surgeon can perform laparoscopic surgery in a number of positions but two main ones exist; between the legs and at the side of the patient. The trainee will find one more ergonomic depending on the procedure. It is usually the surgeon's preference or habit of getting adjusted to a particular position. Subsequent technical steps will vary according to the chosen position. Adopting one or the other position is often necessary to obtain optimal triangulation .

Operating Table Height

The height of operating table should be adjusted between 64 and 77 cm above floor level, depending on the height of the operating surgeon, since the discomfort and operative difficulty are lowest when instruments are positioned at elbow height [10].

Monitor Position

Neck strain can occur with an inadequately positioned monitor. The image should be 25° below the horizontal plane of the eye. It has also been shown that laparoscopic task efficiency can be enhanced if the image is placed near the operative field, adjacent to the hands, because the resultant "gaze-down" view aligns the surgeon's visual and motor axes [10]. A second monitor may be needed for procedures that require position changes or to allow the assistants to see without undue neck strain [11].

Training Situational Awareness (SA)

This subject is fully covered in the Chap. 13 (Human Factors). Surgery, one of the most complicated, time-critical and high-pressure medical practices, demands acute SA. Traditionally, the surgical staff was responsible for monitoring different activities within an operating room. However there are now multiple OR data sources in an operating room and monitoring and analyzing all the data streams arriving from sensors, services and devices can be challenging. Situation awareness simply means understanding the current situation; this requires active involvement and planning.

SA can be trained using a variety of different methods that can be broadly split into theoretical training and virtual reality training. Theoretical training would be a method of discussion with the trainer regarding key points to convey to the trainee. Virtual reality training would employ the use of training simulators in order to assess SA. Tracking (whether eye or instrument) has been shown to be an effective tool (whether eye or instrument) to assess SA.

Training Laparoscopic Skills Inside the OR (Transferring Skills to the Patient)

Most surgical regulatory bodies will have a curriculum that trainees will have to adhere to. This will outline the skills to be attained by the end of a placement and/or year and the number of cases to be completed at various levels of involvement. Trainers should consult with the trainee to help fix realistic goals and also explain what is expected of them as mentors. Inside the OR training will involve equipment learning, trouble-shooting and technical skills attainment. A trainer's method of teaching inside the OR will vary, but should directly relate to the goals set. An evaluation of tasks and skills performed inside the OR should regularly take place, which then provides the focus for learning activities outside the OR. In this way a reciprocal relationship is set up.

Training Safe Access Techniques

When teaching trainees this most elemental step in laparoscopic surgery it is worth bearing in mind that almost fifty percent of all laparoscopic-related major complications occur due to placement of trocars and iatrogenic injury to intra-corporeal structures. The majority of injuries are associated with blind placement of the first trocar or Veress needle, most often but not always at the umbilicus [12, 13].

In addition to the numerous examples of trocar technology available now to the surgeon it is worth remembering that often the most basic teaching methods may yield appropriate and safe results. For instance, resting the trocar inserting hand index finger onto the barrel of the trocar during insertion allows for improved control and decreased likelihood that the trocar will enter an increased depth causing injury. Also, it is important to emphasis that an open-entry technique is associated with a significant reduction in failed entry when compared to a closed entry technique, and is much safer compared to the use of Veress needle [13].

Access can be associated with injuries to the gastrointestinal tract and major blood vessels, and at least 50 % of these major complications occur prior to commencement of the intended surgery. Increased morbidity and mortality result when laparoscopists do not recognize injuries early and/or do not address them quickly. The next step after entry of any trocar into the abdomen is a visual check with the laparoscope to assess any injury to abdominal wall vasculature (bleeding from the internal entry point of the port) and intra-abdominal organ damage. Any such damage should be dealt with immediately and its occurrence clearly indicated in the operation note. The same applies to checking for bleeding during withdrawal of trocars at the end of surgery.

In general, there is no uniform consensus about port placements for laparoscopic procedures. The placement of ports is currently dictated by the type of operation being performed and the surgeons' preference, based on individual experience. For optimal ergonomics and visualization during laparoscopy, trocars are usually placed in a triangular fashion, termed triangulation [14, 15]. The operative field should be fifteen to twenty centimeters from the optical trocar. In general, the remaining trocars (usually two) are placed in the same fifteen to twenty centimeters arc five to seven centimeters either side of the optical trocar. If necessary, retracting ports can be placed in the same arc but more laterally so as to prevent instrument 'fencing' [10].

Grasping

When using graspers it is foremost important to realize there is a lack of visual or haptic feedback. Subsequently, a concentrated increased amount of force may be applied to delicate structures. Appropriate graspers must be applied for the task in hand e.g., atraumatic bowel graspers for handling of bowel.

Hemostasis

Hemostasis, a cornerstone of surgical practice, and has not evolved dramatically in recent times. The principles remain the same and the technology remains based on core principles. Teaching principles and algorithms in the case of bleeding is of the utmost importance. What can be an acute situation requiring awareness can quickly descend into a potential catastrophe if left unattended.

As with many medical principles, prevention is better than cure. The authors note a number of clear principles to help the reader imbue situational awareness and good technique while performing laparoscopic procedures.

1. Clear instrument view at all times within laparoscopic operative field
2. Avoidance of blunt avulsion of structures
3. Pre-division application of coagulation
4. Skeletonization of structures for division
5. Avoidance of potential vascular structures or ligation prior to division.

When hemorrhage occurs, a clear logical process should be followed to ensure it is managed expediently and effectively.

1. Visually identify bleeding area, do not move retraction
2. Use a large bore suction device. Irrigation can obscure the field of view and should therefore be used sparingly. Gauze pads may be inserted in to the intra-abdominal space to tamponade bleeding.
3. Once the bleeding point is identified use an atraumatic or a fine dissecting grasper to control the bleeding
4. If step 3 is successful consider adding more ports to aid retraction if needed.
5. Place a hemostatic clip or clips to control the bleeding but only after you can clearly identify and dissect the bleeding vessel
6. Now use suction irrigation and re-evaluate.
7. If this is unsuccessful, convert to an open procedure

A variety of different methods are available to the surgeon for hemostasis, ranging from direct pressure to novel devices.

Dissecting: Energy Sources (Diathermy, Harmonic Scalpel and Ligasure)

Electro-surgery has revolutionized the art and science of surgery. It has also facilitated laparoscopic surgery due to the enclosed nature of the operative field. The physics of electro-surgery can be found in depth elsewhere and the fundamentals are important when teaching trainees.

The most important point to teach trainees when using energy sources is that the safety of the patient remains paramount. This is extremely important when considering monopolar cautery. Patient electrode pads must be placed in an appropriate position to avoid burns. The patient's skin must not touch metallic objects causing preferential transfer of current through that point, again causing burns.

Once this has been firmly imbued, the position of the electrode tip remains a key component of success in dissection. The second most important component of dissection is the tension and counter-traction obtained by the operator and his/her assistant(s).

Laparoscopy has particular issues with regards to the use of electro-cautery, which the trainee must be made aware of at an early stage, ideally prior to entry into the OR. Nevertheless a recap is often needed. Firstly, as a result of operating in a 'closed' environment i.e., the non-open abdomen, the surgeon may rely on energy devices more than in open surgery. Due to these constraints and the limited view afforded by the camera, bleeding or injury can happen out of the field of view. The magnification of the field of view by modern laparoscopes can make minor bleeding appear greater than it actually is. In spite of the significant advances with laparoscopic surgery, the surgeon still has less tactile feedback and less depth and color perception on the two-dimensional screen compared to open procedures. The tip of monopolar devices must always be kept within the visual field, as activating the device with the tip outside the field of view may cause inadvertent injury. Activation or the tip or the tip simply being hot may cause damage that is not appreciated by the surgeon. This can result in delayed complications. Also many modern instruments do not have complete insulation or there may be the risk of faulty insulation along the shaft. This must be checked regularly by the OR nursing staff. It is the surgeon's responsibility to ensure that the team and the trainee are familiar and trained on using the device before utilization.

Ultrasonic Dissection

Whereas monopolar and bipolar electro-cautery employ electrical energy to produce heat, ultra-sonic devices use vibration to simultaneously cut and coagulate. An example of ultrasonic energy source is the Harmonic Scalpel, which the scalpel blade vibrates 55,500-times per second causing stress and friction in tissue. This in turn generates heat and causes protein welding to allow simultaneously division and coagulation of tissue. The use of this technology is advantageous in as much as dissection times are reduced in addition to less lateral thermal spread when compared to traditional electro-cautery. However, it is important to teach trainees about the heat generated by the ultra-sonic devices, particularly at the tip, which can cause tissue damage [16].

Bipolar Dissectors

This technology employs an electro-surgery generator where the energy is applied across two electrodes. An algorithm detects impedance in the electrical circuit formed and adjusts the energy accordingly until complete coagulation is obtained and then, stopping automatically. This results in an effective welded seal of the tissues. This weld can then be divided without bleeding occurring. Bipolar coagulation instruments are used extensively for coagulation, and have the advantage of being able to grasp tissues at the same time. Other devices exist that combine coagulation and division, such as Ligasure.

Suturing

The authors maintain that incorporeal knot tying is a 'must have' technical skill for all laparoscopic surgeons and thus this skill must be taught to trainees at an early stage. Notwithstanding, intra-corporeal knot tying and suturing remain one of the most difficult and complex techniques performed in surgery.

This technique is best practiced and mastered on a simulator prior to use in the OR by the trainee to reduce operating times [17]. As a key point, the authors hold the needle with the concavity pointed down as to aid in rotation of the needle and hence the thread over and around the non-needle-holding instrument. Bimanual dexterity is paramount to success and sound knotting. The type of suture used will be on the whole similar to as with open surgery, however with the exception of novel laparoscopic suture technology. Suture brands such as V-lock that make it easier to throw sutures without the need for intracorporeal knot tying can be introduced to the trainee at a later stage.

Irrigation/Suction

Irrigation and suction of the intracorporeal cavity can be achieved by insertion of a catheter into usually the 10 mm port. The catheters can be either gravity dependent or powered. The use of irrigation and suction with regards to hemostasis are explained elsewhere in this chapter. Its role in sepsis is less clear. The old adage 'the solution to pollution is dilution', has been heard by trainees during their training to exemplify the use of irrigation where there is pus. The evidence is not as clear-cut, with a recent study showing no advantage of irrigation over suction alone in perforated appendicitis.

As no clear conclusions exist, a individualized approach to each case is still recommended by the authors, encouraging localized pools of pus to be first suctioned rather than irrigated first [18, 19].

Trocar Wound Closure

Port sites greater than 8 mm will need closure with a fascial suture. A technically sound repair is extremely important to teach due to the troublesome complication of port-site hernias, which occur in one to six percent of cases. Techniques to avoid bowel entrapment during the closure should also be taught. The most simple, cheap and effective methods should be taught in the first instance, moving onto more complex methods once the basics have been mastered.

Whatever techniques used (thirty-one have been described to date), a number of key steps need to be incorporated. Protection of the intra-abdominal components to the suture needle is paramount (retractors are most commonly used here) and taking appropriate 'bites' of the fascia to ensure a sound repair must be taught correctly [20–22].

Conclusions

Basic skills are often left aside, as many trainers assume that these are well known to the trainees. In fact, many trainers ignore them as well. A good teacher has the power to inspire, to motivate and to get the very best out of a trainee, not only by example but by good instructing. Teaching basic skills in a focused way with clear goals will pay dividends in the progression of a trainee to an independent practitioner. If basic skills are the core of a solid foundation, we must ensure that those skills taught stand the test of time and change.

References

1. Cameron JL. William Stewart Halsted: our surgical heritage. Ann Surg. 1997;225:445–58.
2. Harackiewicz JME, NJ. The joint effects of target and purpose goals on intrinsic motivation. Pers Soc Psychol Bull. 1998;24:675–89.
3. Locke EAB, J. Goal setting as a determinant of the effects of knowledge of score in performance. Am J Psychol. 1968;81:398–406.
4. Gonzalez R, Bowers SP, Smith CD, Ramshaw BJ. Does setting specific goals and providing feedback during training result in better acquisition of laparoscopic skills? Am Surg. 2004;70(1):35–9. Epub 2004/02/18.
5. McCluney AL, Vassiliou MC, Kaneva PA, Cao J, Stanbridge DD, Feldman LS, et al. FLS simulator performance predicts intraoperative laparoscopic skill. Surg Endosc. 2007;21(11):1991–5. Epub 2007/06/27.
6. Nguyen T, Braga LH, Hoogenes J, Matsumoto ED. Commercial video laparoscopic trainers versus less expensive, simple laparoscopic trainers: a systematic review and meta-analysis. J Urol. 2013;190(3):894–9. Epub 2013/04/10.
7. Sharma M, Macafee D, Horgan AF. Basic laparoscopic skills training using fresh frozen cadaver: a randomized controlled trial. Am J Surg. 2013;206(1):23–31. Epub 2013/04/30.
8. Leblanc F, Senagore AJ, Ellis CN, Champagne BJ, Augestad KM, Neary PC, et al. Hand-assisted laparoscopic sigmoid colectomy skills acquisition: augmented reality simulator versus human cadaver training models. J Surg Educ. 2010;67(4):200–4. Epub 2010/09/08.
9. Joice P, Hanna GB, Cuschieri A. Ergonomic evaluation of laparoscopic bowel suturing. Am J Surg. 1998;176(4):373–8. Epub 1998/11/17.
10. Supe AN, Kulkarni GV, Supe PA. Ergonomics in laparoscopic surgery. J Minim Access Surg. 2010;6(2):31–6. Epub 2010/09/04.

11. Hanna GB, Shimi SM, Cuschieri A. Task performance in endoscopic surgery is influenced by location of the image display. Ann Surg. 1998;227(4):481–4. Epub 1998/05/01.
12. Bhoyrul S, Vierra MA, Nezhat CR, Krummel TM, Way LW. Trocar injuries in laparoscopic surgery. J Am Coll Surg. 2001;192(6):677–83. Epub 2001/06/13.
13. Ahmad G, O'Flynn H, Duffy JM, Phillips K, Watson A. Laparoscopic entry techniques. Cochrane Database Syst Rev. 2012;(2):CD006583.
14. Fingerhut A, Hanna GB, Veyrie N, Ferzli G, Millat B, Alexakis N, Leandros E. Optimal trocar placement for ergonomic intracorporeal sewing and knotting in laparoscopic hiatal surgery. Am J Surg. 2010;200(4):519–28.
15. Manasnayakorn S, Cuschieri A, Hanna GB. Ideal manipulation angle and instrument length in hand-assisted laparoscopic surgery. Surg Endosc. 2008;22(4):924–9.
16. Emam TA, Cuschieri A. How safe is high-power ultrasonic dissection. Ann Surg. 2003;237(2):186–91.
17. Croce E, Olmi S. Intracorporeal knot-tying and suturing techniques in laparoscopic surgery: technical details. JSLS J Soc Laparoendosc Surg/Soc Laparoendosc Surg. 2000;4(1):17–22. Epub 2000/04/20.
18. St Peter SD, Adibe OO, Iqbal CW, Fike FB, Sharp SW, Juang D, et al. Irrigation versus suction alone during laparoscopic appendectomy for perforated appendicitis: a prospective randomized trial. Ann Surg. 2012;256(4):581–5. Epub 2012/09/12.
19. Platell C, Papadimitriou JM, Hall JC. The influence of lavage on peritonitis. J Am Coll Surg. 2000;191(6):672–80. Epub 2000/12/29.
20. Shah PR, Naguib N, Thippeswammy K, Masoud AG. Port site closure after laparoscopic surgery. J Minim Access Surg. 2010;6(1):22–3. Epub 2010/06/30.
21. Hussain A, Mahmood H, Singhal T, Balakrishnan S, Nicholls J, El-Hasani S. Long-term study of port-site incisional hernia after laparoscopic procedures. JSLS J Soc Laparoendosc Surg/Soc Laparoendos Surg. 2009;13(3):346–9. Epub 2009/10/02.
22. Chen K, Klapper AS, Voige H, Del Priore G. A randomized, controlled study comparing two standardized closure methods of laparoscopic port sites. JSLS J Soc Laparoendosc Surg/Soc Laparoendosc Surg. 2010;14(3):391–4. Epub 2011/02/22.

Chapter 5
Training for Trainers in Endoscopy (Colonoscopy)

John T. Anderson and Roland Valori

Abbreviations

DOPS	Direct Observation of Procedure Skills
DOPyS	Direct Observation of Polypectomy Skills
JAG	Joint Advisory Group for Gastrointestinal Endoscopy
TTT	Training the trainers'
TCT	Training the Colonoscopy Trainer
LapCo	TT Laparoscopic colorectal training the trainers
UK	United Kingdom

Background

Training the trainers' (TTT) courses in endoscopy were developed to enhance and spread the expertise of trainers delivering basic and other skills-enhancing courses in endoscopy. The current Training the Colonoscopy Trainer (TCT) course is the most popular format and has become the default TTT course for colonoscopy in Canada, Australia and the UK. The first TCT was delivered in 2003 and has undergone continuous refinement to improve the relevance to colonoscopy and increase

J.T. Anderson, MB ChB, MMEd, FRCP, MD (✉)
Department of Gastroenterology, Cheltenham General Hospital,
Sandford Road, Cheltenham, Gloucestershire GL53 7AN, UK
e-mail: john.anderson@glos.nhs.uk

R. Valori, MB BS, FRCP, MD, MSc, ILTM
Department of Gastroenterology, Gloucestershire Hospitals NHS Foundation Trust,
Great Western Road, Gloucester, Gloucestershire GL1 3NN, UK
e-mail: roland.valori@nhs.net

N. Francis et al. (eds.), *Training in Minimal Access Surgery*,
DOI 10.1007/978-1-4471-6494-4_5

effectiveness and efficiency of training. The TCT course was adapted in 2010 for the English national laparoscopic colorectal surgery training programme (www.lapco.nhs.uk). The resultant LapCo TT (Laparoscopic colorectal training the trainers) course is now an integral part of this programme.

Core Attributes of Effective Trainers

A Trainer Must Be Able to Perform the Procedure Competently

The quality of any medical procedure has a direct impact on the patient. This is particularly the case for colonoscopy where there is evidence that poor quality colonoscopy is more likely to cause complications, be incomplete, be more painful or require excessive doses of sedation and miss and/or incompletely remove important lesions. As a minimum, trainers must be competent in colonoscopy.

Modelling Behaviours

When trainees are deemed competent, they are considered to be safe to perform independently. However, they will, to varying degrees, be performing well short of their potential. To realise potential, particularly in colonoscopy, requires motivation to improve, a conscious approach (active reflection) to identify areas in need of improvement and continuous practice to overcome shortcomings. There is good evidence that trainees model themselves on their trainers, and therefore a second core component of an effective trainer is to set an example of continuously striving to improve performance.

Conscious Competence

Endoscopic expertise encompasses cognitive, behavioural and technical components. To be able to train effectively, a trainer must be able to understand these components and verbalise them – so called *conscious competence*. Explicit knowledge is conscious and can be verbalized. Implicit knowledge is not readily available for conscious recall and difficult to verbalize. Over time highly practiced tasks become automated and experts have less explicit knowledge of their performance compared to novices. For example, most people would struggle to explain clearly the individual stages involved in their limb movement when riding a bicycle. This has been termed "expertise-induced amnesia" and may explain why it is difficult for some experts to explain what they are doing and therefore be able to train others.

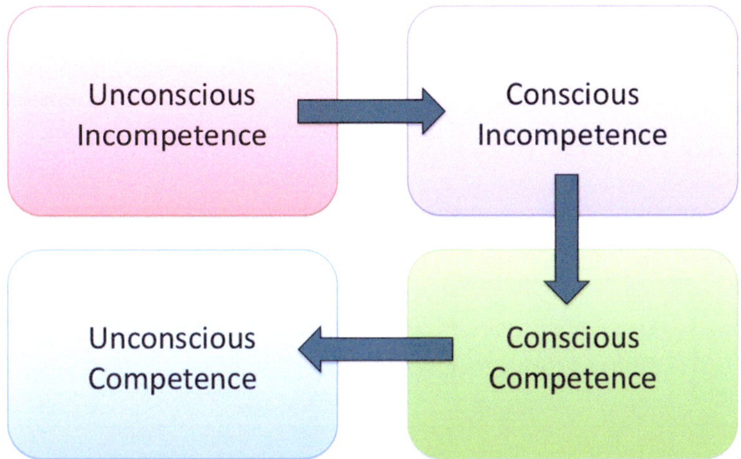

Fig. 5.1 Conscious competence learning cycle

This process has also been noted in the medical education literature. Peyton's learning cycle describes trainees moving from ***conscious competence***, where they can perform a technique but have to think about it, to **unconscious competence** where they have acquired mastery of the technique and no longer have to think about it (Fig. 5.1) [1].

For the majority of trainers, training effectively requires them to move from unconscious competence back a stage to conscious competence. Conscious competence enables explicit deconstruction of the task and the ability to provide explicit explanation of how to successfully complete it. The more novice the trainee, the simpler the deconstruction steps need to be. The individual steps or stages can then be verbalised in an understandable form to the trainee to facilitate learning and skills acquisition.

If trainees understand how the acquisition of a certain knowledge or skill will enable them to perform better, they enter into instructional situations with a clearer sense of purpose and see what they learn as more personal [2].

To train endoscopy effectively requires explicit knowledge of the techniques needed to perform colonoscopy. It also requires explicit knowledge of how to train technical skills. Good trainers need to be consciously competent in both endoscopy and the training techniques to facilitate skill acquisition (Fig. 5.2).

Previous training will influence the ability of individuals to demonstrate conscious competence. The conscious competence phase was frequently bypassed in endoscopy training: trainers acquired skills predominantly through experiential learning. It is a challenge for a trainer who has never been through the conscious competent phase to be able to deconstruct their automated actions. Consequently training of trainees tends to replicate that of the trainers themselves. With increasing understanding of colonoscopy technique, and improved training delivered by consciously competent trainers, trainees, at least in the UK, no longer bypass the conscious competence phase.

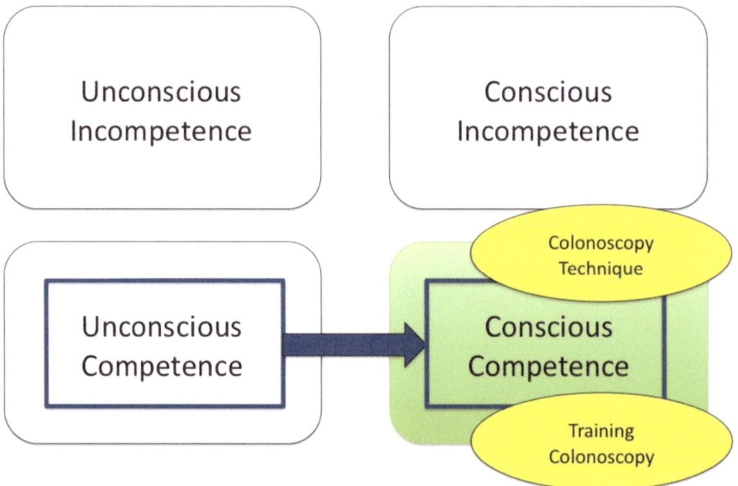

Fig. 5.2 Training effectively: conscious competence of both colonoscopy technique and training skills

Critical Reflection and Analysis

Reflection enables the trainees and trainers to analyse strengths and weakness. Critical reflection is the process where, after reflecting on the whole activity, critical moments are identified for further analysis. In endoscopy training, critical moments are defined as actions or behaviours which lead to either a good outcome (successfully overcoming a difficult problem – to be reinforced), or more commonly, when a trainee struggles in the face of a challenge or difficulty (which often forms the basis for targeted training or feedback). Critical analysis by the trainer is used to promote reflection by the trainee and helps to determine how future actions and behaviours should be modified to improve the outcome when they are encountered again. Core skills a trainer must acquire are the ability to identify critical moments during a procedure, and reflect on these to identify the key learning points.

A Framework for Training Technical Skills

In recent years there has been increasing recognition of the need to train health professionals to teach effectively, but relatively little attention to developing consciously competent technical skills trainers. Bypassing the conscious competence phase of teaching technical skills has two adverse consequences. Firstly, the trainers are less able to develop their own training skills because it is more difficult to self-diagnose what could be done to improve when training does not go well – or even worse, there is failure to recognise when training has gone badly. Secondly, they will be limited in their ability to develop future trainers effectively, similar to the difficulty in trying to train colonoscopy without conscious competence of the procedure.

To help trainers become consciously competent during a training episode it is helpful to deconstruct what constitutes good training. The following section of this chapter uses the **Set** – **Dialogue** – **Closure** framework to deconstruct and then describe the essential components of effective technical skills training. The framework is used in TCT and LapCo TT courses and feedback indicates it is a highly effective approach to teaching technical skills training. The framework provides a set of competencies which trainers can use as a checklist to help then reflect on, and improve their training.

The ***Set*** refers to the period before the commencement of training and can be considered the preparation phase of training. The set has both physical and verbal components. The verbal component should include preparation, assessment of the skill level of trainee, alignment of agendas of both the trainer and trainee and agreement of an educational contract. The physical component of the set relates to the training environment. The trainer should ensure that the environment is designed and set up to facilitate effective training including equipment, ergonomics and position of the trainer.

Dialogue refers to the delivery of the actual training.

Closure is the phase after formal training has been completed. It is in this phase that the trainer should begin to summarise and reflect on the training episode, before facilitating performance enhancing feedback. To complete closure, the trainer agrees with the trainee learning objectives for the next training session.

Components of the Set

The Verbal Set

Effective training requires preparation and structure. In a busy clinical environment preparation time for training is limited. It is important to have a structure to follow to ensure all the key components of preparation are covered.

Assessment

Making a brief assessment of a trainee is particularly important if trainee and trainer have not met before, or if it is some time since the trainer trained a trainee. It is not possible to make a detailed formal assessment of the trainee's skills in the few moments before a training episode. However, it should be possible, with a few well-directed questions, to determine what stage the trainee is at, what particular difficulties they are having and what experience they have. With an e-portfolio this initial assessment is easier and more reliable, particularly if it includes formal competency assessments and learning objectives agreed during the most recent training sessions.

Trainer's and Trainee's Agendas

Trainees often have a concept of what they expect from the training episode (trainee's agenda). If the trainer's agenda differs from this, there is potential for failing to maximise the training opportunity. It is important to determine what the trainees believe they need and adapt to this. If the training episode is driven solely by the trainer, it may deliver effective training, but it will be less well received by the trainee. It is the responsibility of the trainer to be flexible and respond to the challenge of aligning the agendas of trainee and trainer. The learning objectives for each training episode should be a composite of the trainee's and the trainer's agendas [3].

In the early stages of training the trainee is less able to articulate clear goals and objectives – 'they don't know what they don't know'. As training progresses they become much more aware of their training needs, especially if encouraged to critically reflect on their performance. They will then take increasing responsibility for setting learning objectives (Fig. 5.3). Thus a good trainer will encourage the trainee to develop a strong reflective style. This will enable the trainee to achieve the goal of developing responsibility for setting their own learning objectives in an efficient way, when there is no longer a trainer to guide them.

Setting Learning Objectives

If trainees understand how the acquisition of a certain knowledge or skill will enable them to perform better, they enter into instructional situations with a clearer sense of purpose and see what they learn as more personal. In the immediate period

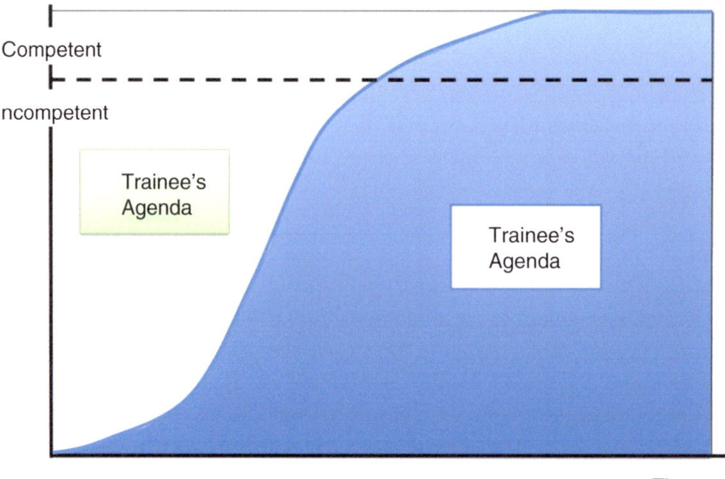

Fig. 5.3 Aligning agendas

before training it is helpful for the trainer and trainee to agree what they will focus on during the procedure or operation – the learning objective(s). Due to the highly variable nature of colonoscopy, it is not always possible for the agreed learning objectives to be addressed and new ones might need to be formulated as the training proceeds.

Educational Contract

An educational contract is an agreement between the trainer and trainee of how they would like the training episode to be conducted [3]. The contract should be agreed before training commences. The processes of assessment, aligning agendas and setting learning objectives form the basis of the contract. In addition, it is important to establish ground rules, such that the trainer and trainee are clear about their respective roles and responsibilities during the training. Most importantly, clear ground rules ensure patient safety, as there will be no uncertainty about who is in control of the procedure and leading the team. Ground rules also establish circumstances in which the trainer might stop the training episode and take over the procedure.

If done effectively, an educational contract enables the trainee to develop their skills and have realistic expectations of what the training can achieve, whilst ensuring the trainer maintains control over the training and the trainee. Creating an educational contract often only requires a few minutes.

The Physical Set

The physical set refers to the positioning of the patient, support staff, equipment, trainee and trainer. Ideally the training environment should be completely free of interruptions and distractions. The intention is to ensure that the environment is safe for patients and staff, but also to ensure the trainee and trainer are as ergonomically comfortable as possible. If sub-optimal, the trainee and trainer may tire or be distracted, and less attention and energy will be directed into the training.

Components of the Dialogue (Instruction and Training)

The dialogue refers to the time from the point the trainee starts the procedure until he/she completes it, or the training episode is terminated.

Instruction during an endoscopic procedure is a critical skill that many trainers find challenging. Having a structured approach facilitates instruction and improves skills acquisition. Conscious competence is a fundamental requirement for effective instruction and without it a trainer will always struggle to make the best of the opportunity. The key aspects of instruction are:

- Specific language
- Type of instruction
- Timing of instruction
- Knowing when to say nothing
- Decision training
- Performance enhancing training
- Training vignettes
- Using competency frameworks

Specific Language

Trainers have, historically, used different words or phrases to explain the same thing. For example, deflect the tip up is the same as turn the big wheel anticlockwise or big wheel down. It is confusing for a trainee to be exposed to different terms for the same action. Instructions directing attention to movement effects are better for enhancing learning than those directing attention to a trainee's arm and hand movements. This may be because directing trainees' attention to an external focus, away from the trainee's hands, allows performance to be mediated by automatic control processes [4]. The implication for training endoscopy is that learning should be improved by instruction focusing on the monitor view, "tip up or tip down" rather than focusing on hand movements, "thumb down or up on big wheel". Anecdotally this approach has proved successful during endoscopic training courses in the UK. It is recommended that directive instruction for colonoscopy be restricted to 12 terms:

1. Stop
2. Pull back
3. Insert
4. Blow
5. Suck
6. Tip Up
7. Tip Down
8. Tip left
9. Tip right
10. Clockwise torque
11. Anti-clockwise torque
12. Slow down/slowly

With these 12 terms or manoeuvres, it is possible to instruct a trainee to insert the instrument safely, ultimately completing the procedure unassisted and in a controlled manner [3]. The completion of this task is dependent on the trainee having the ability to perform the manoeuvres individually and when required, in complex sequences. Washing the lens is an additional term, which may be added to the list, but while clear views are essential, washing the lens does not directly enhance intubation. The use of the words, slowly and stop provides the trainer (and trainee) with increased control over actions and ultimately tip control and problem solving.

Type of Instruction

Broadly speaking instruction can be directive/didactic, or inquisitorial. Asking questions and discussing how to diagnose and solve problems is much the preferred technique. However, for less experienced trainees, or when a more experienced trainee is struggling, a directive approach is more appropriate. The broad types of instruction are as follows:

- Directive: – e.g., deflect the tip up and apply clockwise torque
- Praise: – that was exceptionally well done
- Derogatory: – that was a stupid thing to do
- Observational: – the lumen is at 12 o'clock
- Explanatory: – the luminal view improved because you turned the patient
- Questioning

  Diagnostic: – what do you think is the cause of the problem?
  Solutions: – what are your options for negotiating …………?

A consciously competent trainer will be able to consciously apply these different types of instruction and questioning to best suit the situation. It is hard to justify derogatory or sarcastic comments: they offer no instructional value and they reduce the confidence of the trainee.

Timing of Instruction and When to Say Nothing

As a consequence of cognitive overload trainees may not be able to pay attention to instruction when they are struggling to perform the actual procedure. At these moments it is important for the trainer to keep quiet, providing it is safe for the trainee to proceed. If the trainer needs to instruct, it is better for the trainee to stop the procedure so that he can be fully attentive. Sometimes the trainee has just negotiated a difficult or complex task and is finding it difficult to maintain stability of the instrument. In these circumstances it can be unsettling if the trainer starts instructing. Thus the timing of verbal intervention can be critical. During colonoscopy, even if the trainee is not struggling, it may be appropriate for the trainer to say nothing more than the occasional word of encouragement.

Decision Training

Decision training improves effective decision-making during a task. This is achieved by focusing on critical challenges or problems during the procedure and then choosing the best approach. Decision training has an overt cognitive-motor component and one way it can be employed is by asking questions. In endoscopy it is suggested that if the trainee is unable to make progress, the trainer encourages a diagnosis of the problem and a review of options. The trainer and trainee then agree which options to try and in what order before the trainee resumes scoping. Questions have the benefit of engaging trainees in problem solving and encouraging them to think independently. It improves self-reflection, self-improvement and conscious competence.

Asking questions is an attractive method for improving decision-making but, like verbal commentary, it increases the demands on the trainee. So it seems sensible to restrict questions to when trainees have developed reasonable endoscopic skill, or to stop the procedure to discuss the problem and agree possible solutions. Decision training appears to be most effective for long-term performance at intermediate and advanced levels, and less so for novices.

Cognitive Overload (Dual Task Interference)

Performing two relatively simple tasks concurrently may prove difficult e.g., continuing a conversation while adding up a bill. This phenomenon is known as dual task interference or more specifically 'cognitive overload'. The term cognitive overload is a more accurate term as there are frequently more than two mental processes occurring simultaneously. This phenomenon has been documented across many different fields. The impact of cognitive overload is likely to be due to a bottleneck in mental processing and memory retrieval [5].

Trainees are sometimes encouraged to provide a verbal commentary on their performance. This effectively increases cognitive load and may decrease performance and learning. There are no data to support this method for improving endoscopy skills training. This concept is important, particularly at the start of training and when trainees are struggling and attention demands are highest. In contrast, experts who have developed unconscious competence, have plenty of cognitive capacity for additional tasks such as verbal commentary.

Some training models used in surgical skills training, recommend describing each step *before* it is taken [6, 7]. This type of model may be useful for trainers because it reveals a trainee's decision-making processes and alerts them to potential dangerous actions. However, endoscopy and many other practical skills in medicine are dynamic and it is less easy to describe tasks and actions in a stop-start fashion.

The awareness of the trainer of when a trainee is overloaded with information in relation to the task performance is the key point. If it is important to elicit what the trainee is thinking, questions need to be limited in number and very straightforward to understand. If a more complex discussion is required then it is best to stop the procedure and only restart it when the next steps have been agreed.

In summary, if trainers want to know what trainees are thinking, then asking questions intermittently is preferable to requesting a constant commentary, particularly if the trainee is finding the task difficult.

Performance Enhancing Training

The term *performance enhancing training* brings together all the key components of the dialogue phase of training. This over-arching term includes performance enhancing instruction, performance enhancing feedback, decision training, checking for understanding and other components of effective skills training such as maintaining effective control of training.

Both instruction and feedback can occur before, during or after training, depending on how dynamic the skill is. In some skills such as a tennis serve, events happen too fast to give instruction or feedback during performance of the skill. A tennis player recognizes a poor serve if the ball hits the net, but may not understand what went wrong. A coach watching the same serve can either:

(a) Instruct the player what to do the next time
(b) Help the player understand what he did wrong by asking him, then explaining what happened and discussing how he might improve on this next time

Most endoscopic procedures are slow enough to provide instruction and feedback during the procedure. However, if the trainee is struggling it may not be appropriate to provide <u>either</u> instruction or feedback, because of the impact of cognitive overload.

During endoscopy training, the situation is dynamic and often requires some modification of these educational principles. Dynamic interaction during the procedure could be either instruction or feedback depending on content and context. However, because of the immediate nature of the interaction, this is referred to as instruction, preferably performance enhancing instruction. More didactic instructions are particularly valuable when specifying a clear task goal and when the order in which task components are performed is critical.

Given the nature of endoscopic procedures it is possible to provide the trainee with feedback during the procedure. Feedback delivered in this way should be formative, giving information to a trainee to reinforce or adjust their knowledge, skills and attitudes. Feedback reinforces good performance and addresses areas that require improvement. Emphasizing good practice has a motivating effect and, when feedback is corrective and promotes development, it encourages trainees to modify their behaviour appropriately. Providing feedback concurrently with training has strong immediate performance enhancing effects.

Training Vignettes

There are several common and predictable problems encountered during colonoscopy such as resolving loops, negotiating the flexures and ileal intubation. For each of these challenges it is possible to explain a systematic approach of how to overcome them. It is suggested that trainers develop algorithms or 'training vignettes' for these predictable problems. The process of developing training vignettes improves conscious competence and reduces the negative impact of cognitive overload for the trainer. Having training vignettes to solve predictable problems ultimately makes the procedure more time efficient. This is because the trainer spends less time thinking about how to explain solutions to problems by tapping into a proven, structured approach to resolving the problem.

Components of Closure

Closure refers to the period immediately following a training episode. The aim of closure is to describe and reflect on what happened and then formulate actions (or objectives) for future training episodes. The core of this process is called *performance enhancing feedback*. It is a fundamental component of training which is often overlooked, especially if trainer and trainee consider training to be over when the procedure is finished. When done well, performance enhancing feedback will have a substantial positive impact on the future acquisition of skills.

Performance Enhancing Feedback

Giving feedback after a training episode is an established and effective educational technique, which improves learning considerably [8–10]. Feedback is most effective when it is:

- objective and based on observable behaviours
- given at an appropriate time and place
- expected by the trainee
- given in a non-judgmental way and based on first-hand data
- regulated in quantity and limited to behaviours which are remediable
- a two-way process between the trainer and trainee
- verifiable by the trainee
- specific rather than general
- linked to specific suggestions for improvement

There are several models for giving feedback and no approach is clearly superior to another [11, 12]. A classic model of feedback is the structured approach proposed by Pendleton, which recommends the following steps [13]:

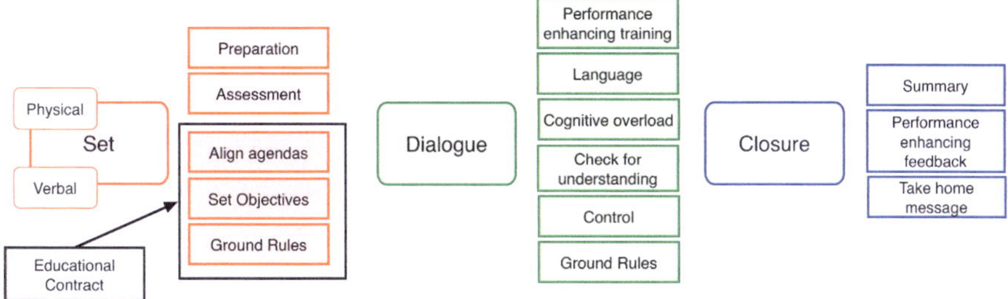

Fig. 5.4 Framework for training practical skills

- The learner goes first and performs the activity
- Questions then allowed only on points of clarification of fact
- The learner then says what they thought was done well
- The teacher then says what they thought was done well
- The learner then says what was not done so well, and could be improved upon
- The teacher then says what was not done so well and suggests ways for improvements, with discussion in a helpful and constructive manner

Unfortunately this approach can feel artificial and contrived, especially if used all the time. The authors apply a more basic structure, which encourages dialogue and exploration of issues in a less structured more flexible fashion. There are three critical steps to this approach (ACT):

1. ***A – Ask the trainee first***: feedback is initiated with an open question asking the trainee what they thought of the training episode with further prompts if the trainee is not forthcoming
2. ***C – Conversation***: there is a conversation between the trainee and the trainer to develop points the trainee raised and any that the trainer wishes to address. The trainer may use a formative assessment tool to inform this conversation
3. ***T – Take home message***: at the end of the feedback there is a clear 'take home' message for the trainee and a specific agreement between the trainee and trainer what the trainee is will do differently – their learning objective(s) – next time to improve their performance.

The conversation between the trainee and trainer is of variable length and detail depending on such factors as context, time available, experience and confidence of the trainee, and the nature of the trainee/trainer relationship. With this approach, the areas that the trainee wishes to focus on are usually discussed first. The trainer must ensure that any reinforcement of good practice is included. This approach is called ***performance enhancing feedback*** to emphasise that the purpose of the feedback is to enhance performance.

The authors have developed a framework for effective efficient delivery of training skills in endoscopy which can be applied to all practical skills training and is summarized in Fig. 5.4.

Other Concepts Contributing to High Quality Skills Training

Scope Handling Techniques Used in Endoscopy Training

There is no evidence that one technique of holding the colonoscope and inserting it is superior to another and widely different techniques are used. In some countries this includes two-person colonoscopy, where one person advances the scope and the other operates the wheels. In endoscopy training it is advised that within a training network one technique of holding and inserting the scope is taught to minimise confusion and accelerate training. Ideally, the technique should be ergonomic, allow precise control and enable the full functionality of the instrument to be available at all times.

Optimal ergonomics are important as an endoscopist often works for long periods, when tiredness and strain injury can reduce performance. Fundamentally, high quality endoscopy is the ability to have very precise control of the instrument at all times. This needs the endoscopist to be able to employ all available and necessary movements of the scope during the entire procedure. From the training perspective the technique should be easy to explain and demonstrate consistently. Once a trainee has been trained to a reasonable level of competence it is not unreasonable for him to be exposed to different methods of holding and manipulating the scope.

Skills Acquisition and Retention

Conditions leading to rapid improvement in immediate performance (acquisition) do not necessarily translate to the same benefits for long-term learning (retention). Anecdotally, trainees attending 'hands-on' endoscopy courses, where they receive intensive instruction and feedback, frequently demonstrate rapid improvements. However, this temporary acquisition effect is not always sustained when the intensive instruction and feedback is subsequently unavailable. For endoscopy, training conditions that improve long-term learning are more important than those, which rapidly improve short-term performance.

After the onset of training an initial rapid rate of learning occurs followed, with practice, by a continued but decreasing rate of improvement [14]. The "10-year rule", supported by studies across such diverse domains as music, chess and sport, suggests that 10 years commitment is needed to acquire expertise [15–17] (Fig. 5.5).

Studies investigating the relationship between volume and competence show learning curves are more gradual than generally appreciated, with numbers required for proficiency being higher than was originally thought necessary and which are currently advised by some organizations and societies [12, 18–21].

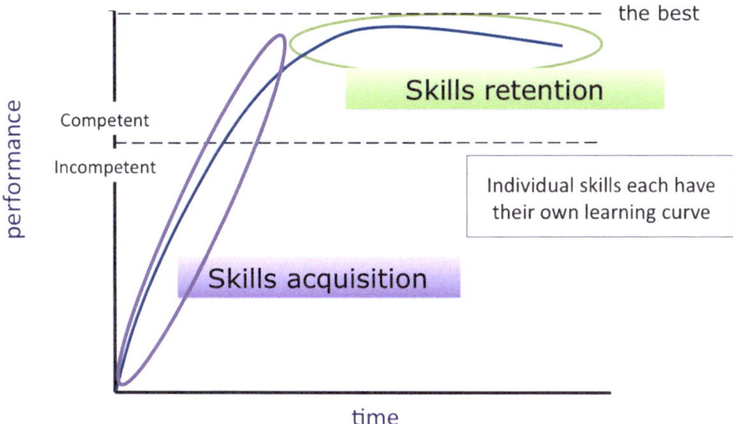

Fig. 5.5 Practical skills acquisition and retention

Practice in Training

'Massed' practice conditions are those where a task is practiced continuously without rest. 'Distributed' practice conditions require rest intervals interspersed with periods of intense practice. Meta-analysis has shown that distributed rather than massed practice conditions are better for both acquisition and retention of skills. However, the optimal rest interval for distributed practice is unknown. A 'distributed' training approach may be more important in the early phases of skills acquisition because the attention load is so great. In practical terms this may mean trainees should not necessarily expect to do all the cases on a training list. There is also some value in observing independent skilled endoscopists, as this can form a blue-print for personal future practice.

Endoscopic Non-technical Skills

Trainees tend to focus on being able to 'complete' a procedure. Once a trainee can perform a complete procedure, they often feel ready to be independent. Prior to independent practice, there is a need to ensure they recognise and can deal with any pathology encountered, as well as anatomical or surgically created variations in anatomy. In addition, there is a requirement to be able to assess mucosa and pathology, make decisions in relation to endotherapy and treatments, and effectively manage and communicate this to the endoscopy team and any other staff involved in the patient's care. These qualities and attributes are known as endoscopic *non-technical* skills. With complete integration of both technical and non-technical skills training, the trainee is more likely to make good judgments and as a result have better patient outcomes and fewer adverse events.

Assessing Competence: Using Competency Frameworks to Enhance Training

Technical skills such as colonoscopy or polypectomy can be deconstructed into component blocks or actions called competencies. Competency frameworks act as a checklist for trainers and a practical guide for trainees. They are used to support training by sign-posting the trainer to areas the trainee needs to focus on to improve. If used appropriately, a competency framework will identify the areas that need to be addressed by the trainer in feedback. Each competency is underpinned by descriptors. The descriptors promote consistency in assessment and scoring; and reduce intra-observer variability. When applied to training, the competency framework enables *formative assessment*: an assessment that supports training. Formative assessment can be applied during the instructional phase of training or during closure when the training is reviewed. A key feature of formative assessment in experiential contexts is that it provides feedback to the trainee with the goal of improving current performance [9].

In the United Kingdom, the formative assessment framework used in endoscopy is called Direct Observation of Procedure Skills or DOPS. There is a specific DOPS for polypectomy called Direct Observation of Polypectomy Skills (DOPyS). Trainers have reported that using the DOPyS to train polypectomy has helped themselves perform better polypectomy as well as making it easier to instruct trainees.

With repeated use, trainers become familiar with the competency framework and no longer find it essential to use them in training: the assessment process becomes automated (unconscious competence) for the trainer. Nevertheless, even when a trainer becomes familiar with the competency framework, the continued use of a competency framework provides both a point assessment and importantly, longitudinal assessment of progress and development of the trainee to competent independent practice. Previous assessments are a useful reference resource for a trainer meeting a trainee for the first time. Ultimately, the competency frameworks may be utilised to provide a summative assessment prior to independent practice.

A key responsibility for trainers is determining when a trainee is competent to perform a procedure independently. The Joint Advisory Group for Gastrointestinal Endoscopy (the JAG) uses the DOPS and DOPyS competency assessment tools, together with performance metrics to determine when a trainee is ready for their final assessment. Details of this process are available on the JAG website (www.thejag.org.uk). The final stage involves a summative assessment using the DOPS on four cases that have to be completed within a set time period. The e-portfolio captures all the relevant information during training attachments and manages the certification process (Fig. 5.6).

For colonoscopy the JAG currently requires a two-stage certification process to full independence. After the first stage the trainee is allowed to practice independently but only with an independent colonoscopist immediately to hand should help

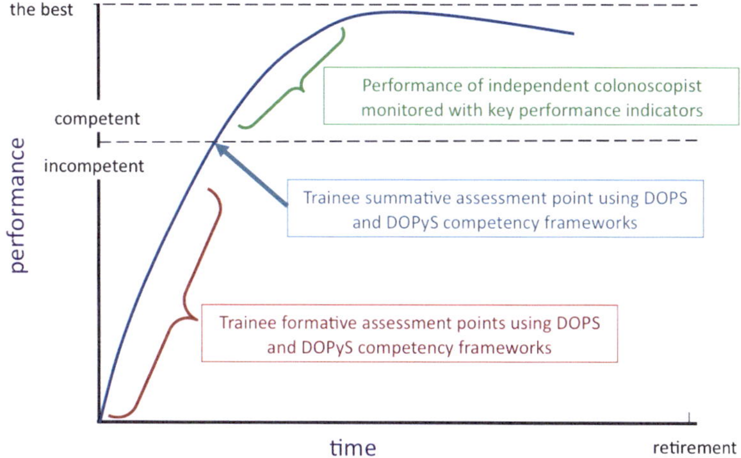

Fig. 5.6 UK Model for assessment of training, certification and on-going practice

be required. Full independence is achieved after submission of competency assessments of polypectomy (DOPyS) combined with a review of performance metrics such as sedation, comfort scores and caecal intubation.

Further Training Beyond Certification

As indicated it is likely to be many years before a colonoscopist achieves their full potential. In our experience review of technique and further training is always valuable regardless of the experience or expertise of the colonoscopist: even highly skilled colonoscopists benefit from development of their conscious competence. Thus we encourage independent trainees and newly appointed consultants to be offered and have further supervised training at regular intervals. Senior doctors will not hesitate to attend conferences and other meetings to keep themselves up to date but will rarely seek further training on their procedural techniques. Trainers should be, and encourage their trainees to become, lifelong learners.

Summary

Endoscopy is a complex psychomotor skill that can be very challenging to teach. Acquiring conscious competence in the procedure is a fundamental step in developing an effective and practical training technique. Education is more about lighting fires than filling buckets, however, using a structured approach (Fig. 5.4) and with application of basic adult learning techniques, training colonoscopy becomes a much more manageable, rewarding and enjoyable experience for both trainer and trainee.

References

1. Peyton J. The learning cycle. In: Peyton J, editor. Teaching and learning in medical practice. 1st ed. Guildford: Manticore Europe Limited; 1998. p. 1–12.
2. Knowles M. The adult learner; a neglected species. 4th ed. Houston: Gulf Publishing Company; P.O. Box 2608, Houston, TX 77001. 1990. p. 128.
3. Anderson J. Teaching colonoscopy. In: Waye JD, Rex DK, Williams CB, editors. Colonoscopy: principles and practice. 2nd ed. New York: Wiley-Blackwell; 2009. p. 141–53.
4. Wulf G, Prinz W. Directing attention to movement effects enhances learning: a review. Psychon Bull Rev. 2001;8(4):648–60.
5. Coderre S, Anderson J, Rostom A, Mclaughlin K. Training the endoscopy trainer: from general principles to specific concepts. Can J Gastroenterol. 2010;24(12):700–4.
6. Walker M, Peyton JWR. Teaching in theatre. In: Peyton JWR, editor. Teaching and learning in medical practice. Rickmansworth: Manticore Europe, Ltd; 1998. p. 171–80.
7. McLeod PJ, Steinert Y, Trudel J, Gottesman R. Seven principles for teaching procedural and technical skills. Acad Med. 2001;76:1080.
8. Ende J. Feedback in clinical medical education. JAMA. 1983;250:777–81.
9. Black P, William D. Assessment and classroom learning. Assess Educ. 1998;5(1):7–74.
10. Vickery A, Lake F. Teaching on the run tips 10: giving feedback. Med J Aust. 2005;183: 267–8.
11. Silverman J, Draper J, Kurtz SM. The Calgary –Cambridge approach to communications skills teaching 2: SET-GO method of descriptive feedback. Educ Gen Pract. 1996;8:16–23.
12. Silverman J, Draper J, Kurtz SM. The Calgary – Cambridge approach to communications skills teaching 1: Agenda led outcome based analysis of the consultation. Educ Gen Pract. 1996;7:288–99.
13. Pendleton D, Schofield T, Tate P, Havelock P. The Consultation: An approach to learning and teaching. Oxford: Oxford University Press. 1984/2003.
14. Newell A, Rosenbloom PS. Mechanisms of skill acquistion and the law of practice. In: Anderson JR, editor. Cognitive skills and their acquisition. Hillsdale: Erlbaum; 1981. p. 1–55.
15. Ericsson KA, Krampe RT, Tesch-Romer C. The role of deliberate practice in the acquisition of expert performance. Psychol Rev. 1993;100(3):363–406.
16. Simon HA, Chase WG. Skill in chess. Am Scientist. 1973;61:394–403.
17. Monsaas JA. Learning to be a world-class tennis player. In: Bloom BS, editor. Developing talent in young people. New York: Ballantine; 1985. p. 211–69.
18. Ward ST, Mohammed MA, Walt R, Valori R, Ismail T, Dunckley P. An analysis of the learning curve to achieve competency at colonoscopy using the JETS database. Gut. doi:10.1136/gutjnl-2013-305973.
19. Koch AD, Haringsma J, Schoon EJ, et al. Competence measurement during colonoscopy training: the use of self-assessment of performance measures. Am J Gastroenterol. 2012;107: 971–5.
20. Spier BJ, Benson M, Pfau PR, et al. Colonoscopy training in gastroenterology fellowships: determining competence. Gastrointest Endosc. 2010;71:319–24.
21. Wexner SD, Litwin D, Cohen J, Earle D, Ferzli G, Flaherty J, Graham S, Horgan S, Katz BL, Kavic M, Kilkenny J, Meador J, Price R, Quebbemann B, Reed W, Sillin L, Vitale G, Xenos ES, Eisen GM, Dominitz J, Faigel D, Goldstein J, Kalloo A, Peterson B, Raddawi H, Ryan M, Vargo J, Young H, Simmang C, Hyman N, Eisenstat T, Anthony T, Cataldo P, Church J, Cohen J, Denstman F, Glennon E, Kilkenny J, McConnell J, Nogueras J, Orsay C, Otchy D, Place R, Rakinic J, Savoca P, Tjandra J, American Society for Gastrointestinal Endoscopy, Society of American Gastrointestinal Endoscopic Surgeons, American Society of Colorectal Surgeons. Principles of privileging and credentialing for endoscopy and colonoscopy. Gastrointest Endosc. 2002;55(2):145–8.

Chapter 6
Teaching Advanced Laparoscopic Skills in Colorectal Surgery

Slawomir Marecik and Roberto Bergamaschi

Introduction

For more than 100 years, the teaching of surgical skills has been performed using the apprenticeship model of graded responsibility, introduced by William Halsted. Over the years, this approach of "see one, do one, and teach one" has been successfully used to train generations of surgeons in all aspects of open surgery [1].

Today, however, the introduction of laparoscopic surgery and the development of more advanced laparoscopic procedures have shown that this well-tried method of teaching is no longer the ideal model for laparoscopic surgery. This is largely due to the recognition that laparoscopic surgery requires the development of an entirely different set of skills. As a result, there is now need to change the existing system of surgical training [2, 3].

Acquisition of Basic Laparoscopic Skills

The unique features that have made laparoscopy the method of choice for many surgical procedures are the same factors that have necessitated the acquisition of a new, different set of skills. These include the fulcrum effect of the instrument in the

S. Marecik, MD, FACS, FASCRS
Division of Colorectal Surgery,
Advocate Lutheran General Hospital, University of Illinois MC,
1775 Dempster Ave., Park Ridge, IL 60068, USA
e-mail: smarecik@uic.com

R. Bergamaschi, MD, PhD, FRCS, FACS, FASCRS (✉)
Division of Colorectal Surgery, State University of New York,
HSCT 18, Room 051, SUNY Stony Brook, Stony Brook, NY 11794-8191, USA
e-mail: rcmbergamaschi@gmail.com

N. Francis et al. (eds.), *Training in Minimal Access Surgery*,
DOI 10.1007/978-1-4471-6494-4_6

trocar, decoupling of the surgeons eyes and hands by an independent camera, changed depth perception of the two-dimensional image, modified haptic feedback, often needed ambidexterity, stereognosis, different exposure techniques, and ergonomics [2, 4].

The number and complexity of laparoscopic procedures, many factors play a role in skill-acquisition. Among them are costs and time constraints. Additionally, because the actions of the trainee cannot easily be controlled by the trainer, as with the open technique, errors can occur that may cause harm to the patient. Thus, it is critical for surgeons to learn these motor skills by more than just passive observation and dismiss the notion that laparoscopic skills can be learned simply by holding the camera [5]. Some have even predicted that robots will eventually steer an independent camera for the surgeon [6] (Fig. 6.1).

Also impacting on the acquisition of these new skills are recent regulations put into place to ensure shorter duty hours for surgical residents. While important, there is concern that reduced basic and advanced laparoscopy training in the surgical residency curriculum could lead to a deficiency in laparoscopic training, placing patients at additional risk for injury.

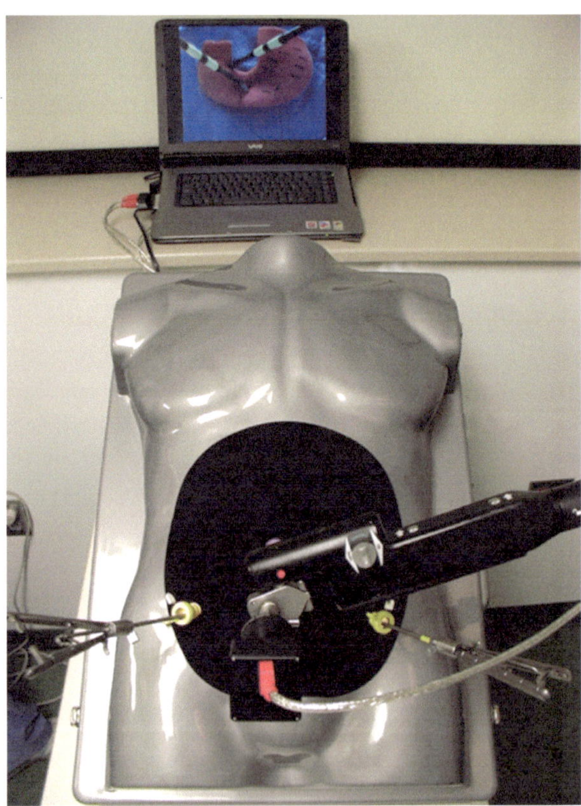

Fig. 6.1 Robotic arm stearing the camera

Simulation, Skill Labs and Video Analysis

Training outside of the operating room offers a structured and systematic educational opportunity, in addition to stress modulation. Because the operating room is a stressful place with many distractions, time constraints, concerns for the patient, equipment failures, and interpersonal issues [7, 8], stress modulation was found to enhance performance when fine motor control and complex cognition are required [9].

The effectiveness of simulation has been demonstrated primarily in lower level learners [10]. According to Fitts and Posner, the first two stages of motor skills acquisition can be sufficiently accomplished in simulation labs. These include the cognitive stage (intellectualization of the task) and the integrative (associative) stage (translation into appropriate motor behaviour), which are achieved by practice and feedback. Accomplishing both stages allows one to proceed to the third stage, the autonomous stage, which is mastered in the operating theatre and results in a smooth performance without cognitive awareness [11, 12].

Today, multiple models of simulation are available, though there is no consensus on which dexterity drill should be incorporated into simulation models for the acquisition of appropriate motor skills [2]. As pointed out by Aggarwal et al that it is not a matter of which simulator to use to acquire the skill, but rather the design of the laboratory-based skills training curriculum [13]. Trainees can evaluate their own performance by comparing their results to the standards associated with a particular simulator, and then working to minimize the difference with subsequent exercises (internal feedback). The use of expert evaluators is also important as they can provide external feedback to the trainees, including information about effectiveness and quality of the operating end product (Fig. 6.2). Procedure effectiveness can be evaluated using an objective assessment of various outcome measures, including goal and non-goal directed actions, forces and torques, operating time, etc. The quality of the operative end product can then be assessed by the end product analysis, which includes accuracy, error, tissue damage (e.g. water tightness of anastomosis) and with the histological outcome (total mesorectal excision for instance).

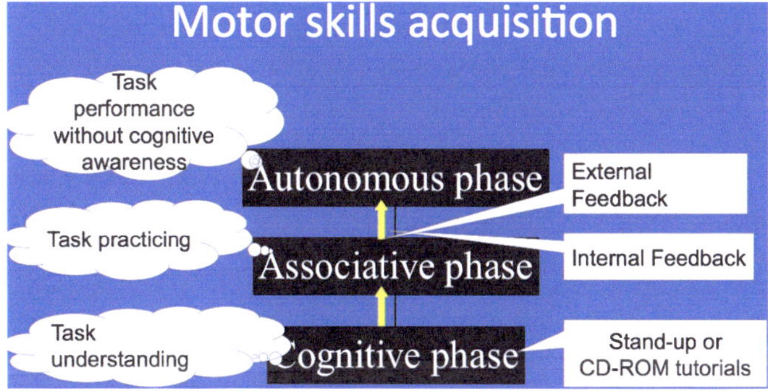

Fig. 6.2 Motor skills acquisition process

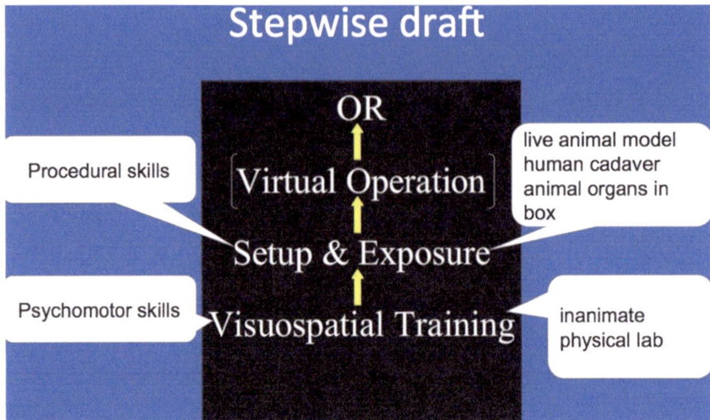

Fig. 6.3 Stepwise approach to learning complex surgical skills

External feedback was found to be critical to the learning process [2, 14, 15]. In particular, summary expert feedback, which takes place after completion of the task, was found to be more efficacious than concurrent feedback, which occurs during completion of the task [16]. It has been reported that there is poor correlation between the procedure effectiveness and the end product analysis [17]. This indicates that a range of pattern of movements during the exercise can result in a similar quality of end product. Interestingly, the end product quality was not adversely affected by the surgeon's fatigue [17]. However, this was investigated on simulated task on VR and it would be interesting to see the correlation between the quality of complex surgery such as laparoscopic total mesorectal excision and the end product. The end product analysis has also been found to be suited for skills assessment, despite its low reliability [2].

Deliberate practice is one of the components of the integrative (associative) phase of motor skills acquisition. It is most effective when distributed throughout many sessions, as opposed to one long single session, because the intervals between sessions allow knowledge of the new skill to be consolidated [18].

For simulation to be successful, the training must be recreated outside of the operating room for all students of surgery, including those with basic as well as advanced skills. A simulated learning environment can be easily controlled and adjusted to varying levels of difficulty. It can also occur in a more step-wise fashion than one performed in the operating room, where learning relies on random chance and opportunity [8] (Fig. 6.3) The step-wise model for learning a complex surgical procedure is based on the premise of building skills gradually using previous accomplishments, with more advanced skills built on a foundation of basic skills. Every complex surgical procedure can be broken down into several simple tasks that are required to complete most complex operations [19]. One of the first teaching modules for laparoscopic surgery was created by Rosser et al. and involved three basic task stations to teach a two-handed technique, coordination in handling tissue and manipulation of a sewing needle [20].

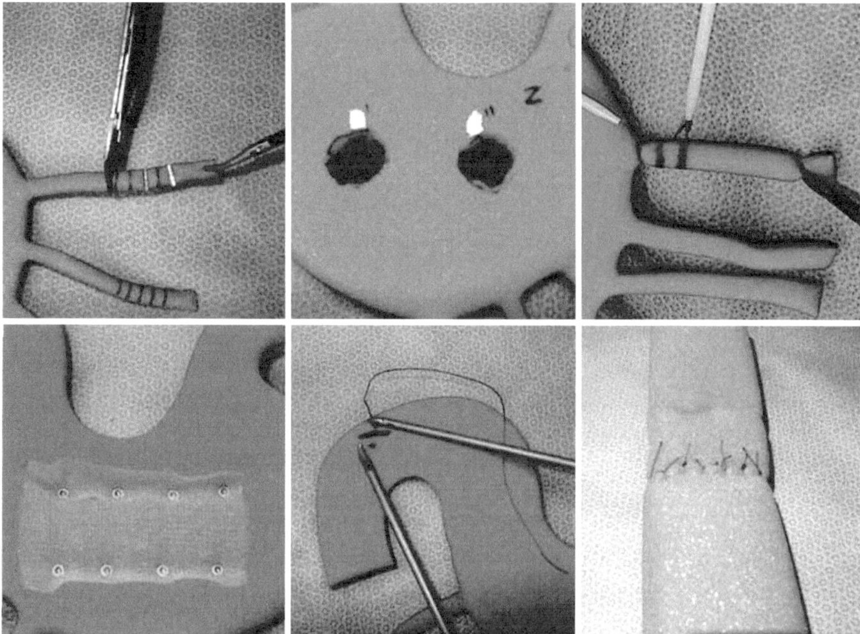

Fig. 6.4 Clinically significant exercise models

Further evolution of the programme led to abandoning the simplified peg exercise program and validating clinically significant exercise models, including vascular control, lesion excision, appendicectomy, mesh repair, perforation closure, and hand-sewn anastomosis [21]. (Fig. 6.4) The basic task analysis and its performance is the first step in the step-wise model of learning the complex surgical tasks. The second step of this process is frequently performed concurrently with the first step, and is often unrecognized. Called visual-spatial training, this step places emphasis on a three-dimensional relationship of anatomic structures and surgical manoeuvres and stresses the importance of proper knowledge of the key relationships of vital structures and dynamic anatomy during an operation. While building on these skills, the trainee can then proceed to the third step, which is practice of the set up and exposure (Fig. 6.3) Interestingly, this step is also under-appreciated by trainees, but valued by experts. In fact, mastering the art of set up and proper exposure enables the surgeon to avoid struggling with poor ergonomics and insufficient exposure during laparoscopic procedures. The sequential steps of the operation become much easier when a proper set up is used [8].

The final step in the step-wise model is the procedural component. Ideally, the student should be able to practice and master the full procedure in the controlled simulated setting. Additionally, while the first three steps can be accomplished with the use of low fidelity simulators, the fourth step can be accomplished with high fidelity inanimate physical models, virtual reality simulators, or cadavers. The procedure should be performed repeatedly in the simulated environment until proficiency

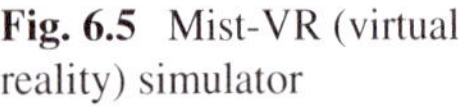

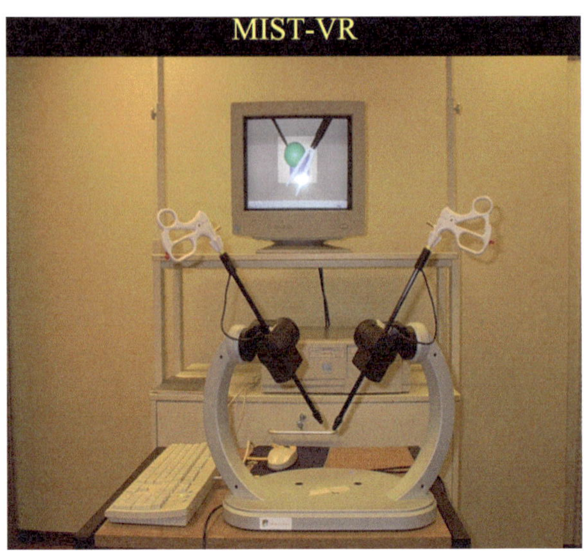

Fig. 6.5 Mist-VR (virtual reality) simulator

is achieved. The term isoperformance was introduced by Jones to describe how learning by two different methods will transfer the same skills, albeit with different efficiency [22]. It is also important to remember that surgical training will always require operating on a real patient, thus the presence of thoughtful mentors to guide the trainee is essential. In fact, technical proficiency is only a single component of the mix; simulation enables the trainee to focus more on the other aspects of the "mix" during clinical exposure, such as obtaining higher-level skills to learn more complex steps of the operation or how to manage complications [8, 23].

Inanimate physical models, including box trainers and bench models, are safe, portable, reproducible, accessible, and readily accepted by novice trainees. They offer a low-fidelity environment for practicing basic, discrete skills and tasks, but not full operations [21]. They also provide true haptic feedback and allow the acquisition of skills that are transferable to complex laparoscopic tasks [24]. Together with the web-based study guidelines, the use of inanimate physical models has been incorporated into the curriculum of the FLS (Fundamentals of Laparoscopic Surgery) programme, endorsed by the American College of Surgeons and the Society of American Gastrointestinal and Endoscopic Surgeons [25, 26]. One of the main advantages of the inanimate physical model is the ability to exercise the dynamic coupling of hands, eyes, and the interposed camera, a skill that is crucial in the operating theatre and not achievable using virtual reality simulators [27]. Sroka et al. found that training to proficiency using the FLS simulator in the surgical residency curriculum has resulted in improved resident performance in the operating room [28].

Virtual reality (VR) simulators, for which the setup time is minimal can provide immediate feedback and metrics on error rates, precision, and accuracy [29]. The identification and subsequent management of errors is crucial to safe surgical practice [30]. Grantcharov et al. was able to detect a higher economy of motion and fewer errors while performing laparoscopic cholecystectomy, as well as shorter operative time after using the MIST-VR simulator [31] (Fig. 6.5). This has been

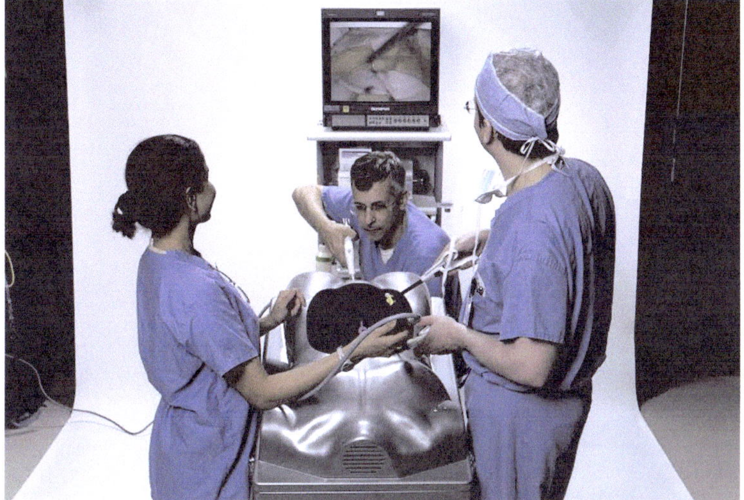

Fig. 6.6 Hybrid ProMIS simulator with synthetic anatomical trays and VR metrics

confirmed by others [32]. One of the disadvantages of the high-fidelity VR simulator is the cost, though this can be outweighed by the benefits. Additionally, one has to remember that surgical training without use of a simulator is associated with significant expense. Bridges and Diamond investigated the cost of having general surgery residents present in the operating room and estimated the annual cost to be $53 million in the United States in 1997 [33]. Conversely, Aggarwal et al. calculated the transfer effectiveness ratio of a modestly expensive VR simulator to be 2.28 for laparoscopic cholecystectomy, translating into every hour spent on VR simulation, and reducing time to achieve proficiency in vivo by 2.3 h [34], thus limiting the costs of training in the operating room.

More recently, the high-fidelity environment was reproduced using the hybrid ProMIS simulator with synthetic anatomical tray and VR metrics (Fig. 6.6). Precise time measurement, instrument path length, and smoothness of movements can all be recorded for analysis [35]. A study comparing the ProMIS simulator with the cadaver model for laparoscopic left colectomy found that technical skills acquisition was better using the simulator. The main overall occurrence in both models was error in the use of retraction, while the specific occurrence in both models was bowel perforation [36]. Essani et al. found that simulated laparoscopic sigmoidectomy training affected the responsiveness of surgical residents with significantly decreased operating time and anastomotic leak rate [37] (Figs. 6.7, 6.8 and 6.9) Another report, however, found no correlation between the simulator-generated metrics (path length, smoothness of movements) and the content valid outcome measures (accuracy error, knot slippage, leak or tissue damage) [38] (Fig. 6.10).

Animate models (porcine and canine), have also been used in training to enable the trainee to practice on live animals, experience the quality of live tissues, and address haemostasis. Apart from ethical considerations, the main obstacles or deficiencies of this model are the differences in anatomy and the need for technical support.

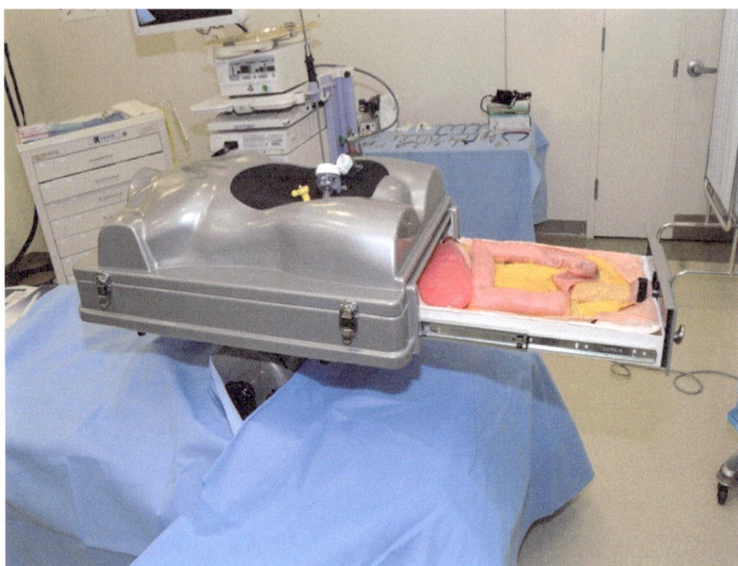

Fig. 6.7 Synthetic anatomical tray of ProMIS simulator

Other options include human cadaveric models, which more closely reflect reality. Milsom et al. performed one of the first feasibility studies of cadaveric laparoscopic proctosigmoidectomy in 1994, designing a standardized technique of oncologic resection [39]. Studies have found participants in cadaver laboratories to be highly satisfied with the teaching value and reliability of the materials used [40, 41]. The main advantages of a cadaveric model include tissue consistency and preservation of anatomic planes, which are very important for the learning process [42]. Le Blanc et al. compared human cadavers and augmented-reality simulators for acquisition of laparoscopic sigmoidectomy skills, finding cadavers to be more difficult but better appreciated than the simulators [36]. Human cadavers were also found to be superior in laparoscopic colectomy training when compared to high-fidelity virtual reality simulators [43]. A recent study reported that colonoscopy training with deployment of stents for colonic strictures in a cadaver model has content, construct and concurrent validity [44]. The major difficulties encountered with cadaver models include their limited availability, high cost, ethical concerns, need for specialized facilities and personnel, andthe inability to exercise haemostasis.

Video analysis is one of the least examined and least understood training methods in laparoscopic surgery. This is ironic because laparoscopic surgery is often referred to as video surgery. In fact, use of a recording device in the operating room is almost a universal standard today. With video analysis, the trainee has the opportunity to review the recorded material individually or with the trainer, who can then provide the necessary critique. Additionally, material can be stored for future use as a reference tool during independent practice, particularly during a low case volume

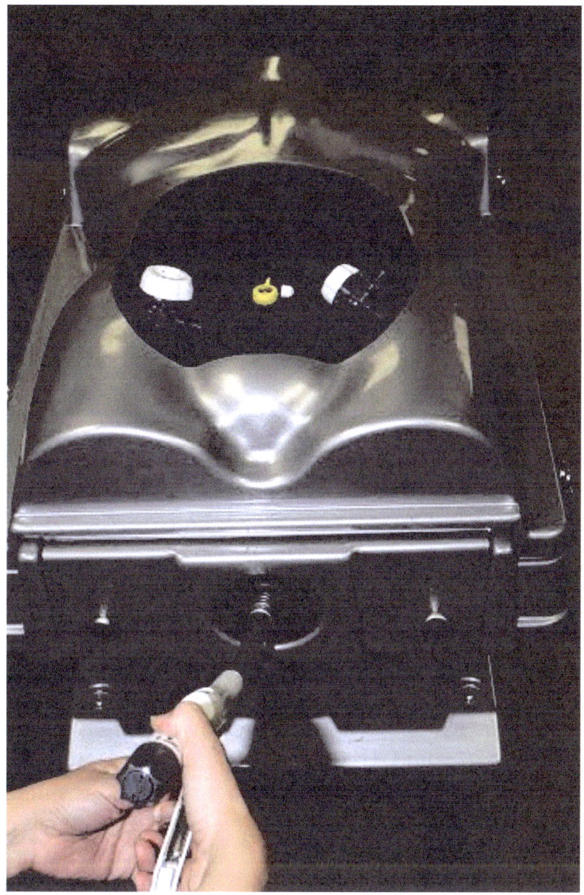

Fig. 6.8 Circular stapling performed with ProMIS simulator

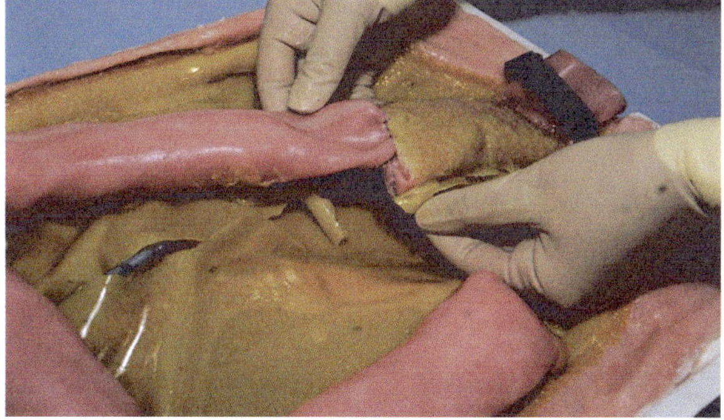

Fig. 6.9 End result of stapling (ProMIS simulator)

schedule. Recorded material can be also used for grading and progress evaluation of the trainee. Ideally, review of the video should take place within a few days (preferably 1–2) of the procedure being performed, so that it is still fresh in both the trainee's and trainer's memory and the intra-operative comments can be remembered.

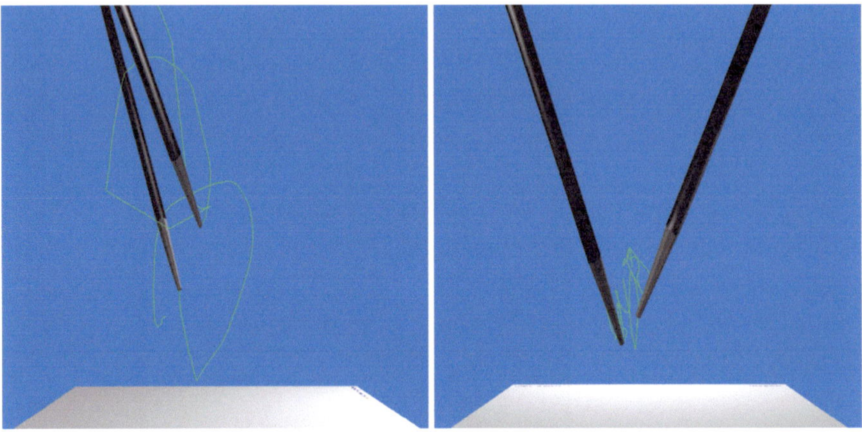

Fig. 6.10 Simulator registered instrument movement path

In 2008, a systematic review of randomized and non-randomized data by Sturm et al. was inconclusive as to which skills learned during laparoscopic simulation were transferable to the operating theatre [45]. More recently, however, Sroka et al. was able to demonstrate that skills learned from the FLS program improved performance during laparoscopic cholecystectomy [28]. Likewise, a systematic review by Zendejas et al. of simulation-based laparoscopic surgery training was found to have significant benefits when compared with no intervention, and moderately more effective when compared to non-simulation intervention (e.g. video instruction) [46]. Despite the validation of many inanimate and VR simulators, there is only one study demonstrating a direct effect of simulation on improved performance in colorectal surgery. In the study by Palter and Grantcharov, a comprehensive curriculum consisted of a VR simulator, a cognitive training component and cadaver lab training. The curricular-trained residents were found to demonstrate superior performance during right colectomy when compared with conventionally trained residents [47].

Little is known about teaching the new techniques of colon resection with single-incision laparoscopic surgery (SILS) or natural orifice trans-luminal endoscopic surgery (NOTES). The only available report by Buscaglia et al. examined the usage of ProMIS simulator for training in NOTES sigmoidectomy, demonstrated a positive outcome for surgical endoscopists with a 42 % reduction in operating time [48] (Figs. 6.11, 6.12, 6.13 and 6.14).

Implementation of Laparoscopic Colorectal Surgery

According to recent reports, the use of laparoscopy in colorectal surgical procedures is gradually increasing, although it has been a very slow process, with varying adoption rates. In 2009, 50 % of all colon resections in the United States were performed laparoscopically [49]. This was up from 31.4 % in 2008, as reported by

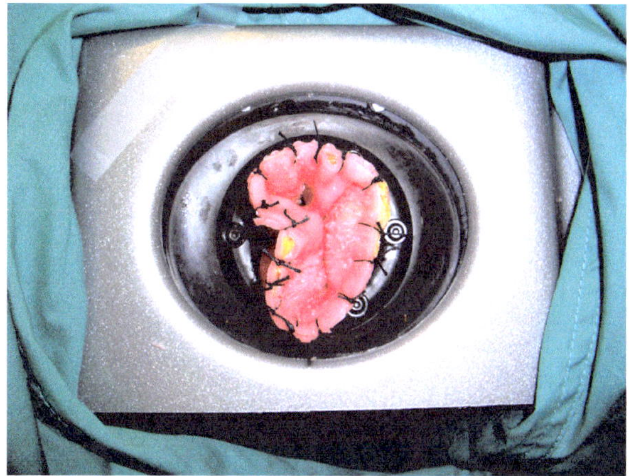

Fig. 6.11 Natural orifice transluminal endoscopic surgery (NOTES) on ProMIS simulator

- 1. Endoscopic viscerotomy with balloon.
- 2. Endoscopic incision and dissection of retroperitoneum.
- 3. Endoscopic identification of left ureter, clipping and transection of inferior mesenteric artery and vein.
- 4. Transanal insertion of second colonoscope.
- 5. Endoscopic mobilization of splenic flexure.
- 6. Endoscopic mobilization of left colon and rectum.
- 7. Endoscopic intussusception of specimen and eversion of rectum with extracorporeal transection of proximal margin at viscerotomy site.
- 8. Hand sewn colorectal anastomosis.

Fig. 6.12 Procedural steps for NOTES sigmoidectomy on ProMIS simulator

a different study only a year before [50]. Similarly, in the United Kingdom, laparoscopy was used in more than 40 % of all colectomies performed in 2013 (according to Hospital Episode Statistics) compared with 5 % of procedures performed in 2006.

Many factors are responsible for these increased adoption rates. During the early adoption phase of laparoscopy, there were concerns about oncological safety, due to reports of trocarsite recurrence [51]. This issue was subsequently eliminated with appropriate wound protection, tissue handling, and proper oncological dissection. Other factors responsible for slower adoption included the need for multi-quadrant dissection, advanced laparoscopic techniques (for intra-corporeal vessel control, large surface dissection, bowel transection, and anastomosis), difficult retraction and exposure, increased operating time, and the cost of the laparoscopic equipment.

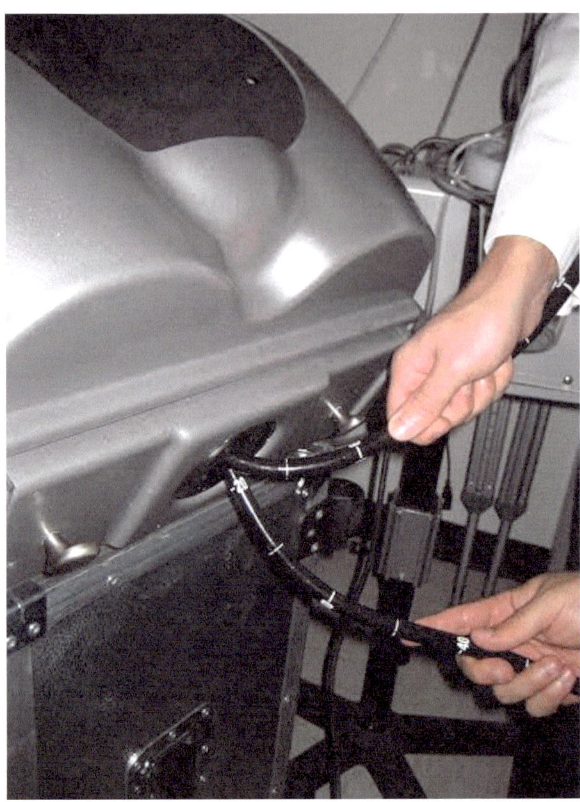

Fig. 6.13 NOTES sigmoidectomy on ProMIS simulator using 2 flexible instruments

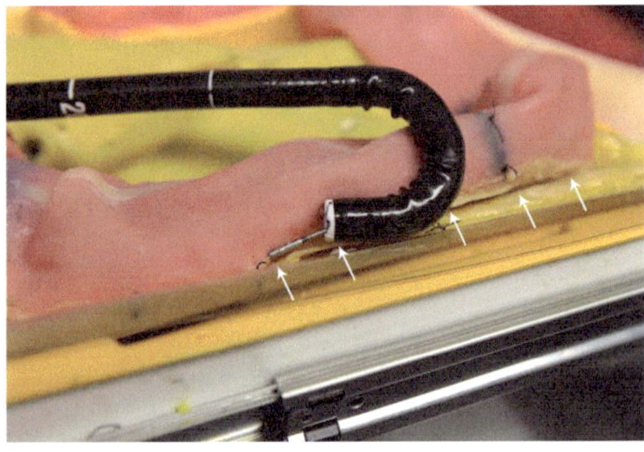

Fig. 6.14 NOTES sigmoidectomy on ProMIS simulator using 2 flexible instruments

The implementation of laparoscopic rectal dissection has been even slower than with colectomy. This is due mainly to tumour location within the rigid confines of the pelvis, difficult and unstable retraction, visualization, and poor ergonomics for the surgeon. In 2009 laparoscopic total mesorectal excision ranged from 12 % in the United Kingdom to 19.6 % in Canada and 26 % in Australia in 2008 [52, 53].

Identification of Trainees

When considering potential candidates for laparoscopic colorectal surgery training, three groups should be identified. The first group is general surgery residents who possess basic laparoscopic skills, but are in the process of acquiring colorectal knowledge and advanced laparoscopic skills simultaneously, in order to perform colectomies. The second group is individuals who are trained in general surgery and are undergoing postgraduate training (colorectal surgery or minimally invasive surgery training). This group is adept in the basics of laparoscopy and has sufficient colorectal knowledge, but lacks experience with laparoscopic colectomies. Finally, the third group is surgeons who have never been trained in laparoscopy but have sufficient experience in open colorectal surgery.

Identifying to which group the trainee belongs is critical and will determine which training model is the most suitable for the trainee. As a result of the time constraints of surgical training mentioned earlier, the first group of trainees is likely to be able to complete only basic training in laparoscopic colectomy. Indeed, unless they engage in postgraduate training, it is unlikely that they will become proficient in advanced laparoscopic colectomies or rectal resections. Conversely, the second group of trainees, because they are involved in postgraduate training (colorectal surgery residents or minimally invasive fellows), is capable of developing the full set of advanced skills required for advanced colectomies and rectal dissection. For the third group, it is expected that they will achieve the same set of skills as the first group, albeit through a different training path.

Regardless of the group, it is important to realize that each is comprised of individuals with different learning potential and, thus, will require individual learning curves.

Learning Curve, Proficiency Gain, and Competence

One of the primary reasons behind the slow adoption of laparoscopy into colorectal surgery has been referred to as a "steep learning curve". However, this description of the learning process is not valid for two reasons. Firstly, the term "learning curve" should be replaced by "proficiency-gain curve", which more accurately describes the process of increasing levels of technical and non-technical proficiency, rather than simply 'learning', which implies a purely cognitive process [54]. Secondly, the term "steep" is a misnomer because it implies rapid acquisition of skills during the time period, quite contrary to what is observed in practice. Therefore, it is more accurate to reason that a "long proficiency-gain curve" is why the adoption process of laparoscopic colorectal surgery has been slower.

There have been many metrics used to describe the learning (proficiency-gain) curve of laparoscopic colorectal surgery. The most commonly used metrics include operative time, conversion rate, complication rate, and readmission rate [55–57].

The main limitations of these individual metrics, however, are their non-transferability throughout different hospitals and individual surgeons [58]. A recent systematic review and multi-centre analysis of multiple metrics, utilizing the risk adjusted CUSUM methods performed by Miskovic et al. estimated the learning curve in laparoscopic colorectal surgery to be between 88 and 152 cases [59]. This number differs from 60 found by Tekkis et al. in 2005 and is in sharp contrast to the range of 11-15 cases identified by Simons et al. in 1995 [57, 60]. This discrepancy can likely be explained by the increasing complexity of the laparoscopic procedures and the application of laparoscopy to more challenging clinical scenarios. Recently, Mackenzie et al .looked at the influence of mentored training on the proficiency-gain curve. They found that 40 cases were required in order for supervised fellows to achieve confidence in laparoscopic colectomy [61].

Monitoring and Assessing the Learning Process

The goal of every training programme is to produce a competent trainee who can individually perform procedures in a safe manner. This competency is difficult to measure prospectively. Indeed, the ultimate method of evaluation used to be the retrospective analysis of clinical outcomes, which were often negative, and included mortality and morbidity data. It is important to recognize that competence is multi-factorial and dependent on surgical skills, cognitive factors, personality traits, and decision-making [62].

The proficiency gain should be closely monitored during the training period. Thus far, various tools have been utilized, including the OSATS (Objective Structured Assessment of Technical Skills). Unfortunately, the value of this tool in the assessment of advanced laparoscopic procedures (e.g. colectomies) has been restricted, due to the ceiling effect and the learning curve of the assessor [63]. The Global Assessment Score (GAS) tool on the other hand, has been found to effectively assess and monitor the proficiency gain. This tool evaluates generic task steps for laparoscopic colorectal resection in a formative way, allowing for the identification of areas during the operation that may be more difficult to master and thus require more practice [64]. Another tool designed to evaluate technical competency in a summative manner is the Competency Assessment Test (CAT). Designed by a reiterative expert consensus (Delphi) method, the CAT evaluates the process of performance (instrument use, tissue handling) as well as the end product of the procedures. It has been validated for examining and credentialing use [65].

While maintaining competency is crucial, little has been made available with regard to the individual retention of learned skills. In fact, while institutions with higher case volumes have shown improved outcomes, some argue that it is the number of hours spent on deliberate practice by the individual surgeon that ultimately determines the level of expertise [66, 67]. However, others contend that tracking outcomes is likely to be the only reliable way to assess competency [68].

Safe and accurate operating can also be assessed using the observational clinical human reliability analysis (OCHRA). This concept, proven in other laparoscopic procedures, is based on video analysis of errors made during procedures and allows for identification of underlying performance-shaping factors [69].

Standard Training Models

Apprenticeship, General Surgery

In Europe and in the United States, the general surgery training system is based on a graded responsibility model in the form of a rotation schedule. The trainees rotate through a designated service (e.g. colorectal or general surgery) for a limited amount of time and receive their training from a qualified trainer (apprenticeship model). On average, surgery residents receive the bulk of their laparoscopic colorectal experience during a 2-month rotation in the 4th year of the 5-year residency program in general surgery. It is during that short period of time that the trainee is expected to participate in 15–30 laparoscopic colectomies. However, additional training in laparoscopic colorectal surgery will take place during a 1-year fellowship in colorectal surgery for those who choose to achieve subspecialty certification ".

The trainee is expected to achieve basic training in laparoscopic colorectal procedures with particular emphasis on safety during such a short period. It is unlikely that proficiency can be fully achieved during such a short period of time. Advanced procedures such as intra-corporeal anastomosis or laparoscopic total mesorectal excision should not be the training goal during this phase of learning.

Dedicated Fellowships and Postgraduate Training in Advanced Laparoscopy

Currently, fellowship training in colorectal surgery with an advanced laparoscopic component, or dedicated minimal access surgery fellowship with a strong colorectal component are considered the ideal and are the most comprehensive forms of training to obtain proficiency in advanced laparoscopic colorectal procedures. These fellowships typically last 1 or 2 years and, and on average, the training program is structured in the form of an apprenticeship. Supervision allows for a shorter proficiency-gain curve and the substantial time period allows the trainee to be exposed to a variety of surgical procedures, including intra-corporeal anastomosis and laparoscopic total mesorectal excision. While for the majority of trainees, fellowships are the continuation of general or specialty training, some surgeons find it difficult to commit to a fellowship, due to the potential impact on their practice and income. However, Schlachta et al. found that within the first year of practice, fellowship-trained surgeons had conversion rates equal to experienced surgeons [70].

Master Class, Short Courses

Master classes or short courses in laparoscopic colorectal surgery are offered as 2 to 7-day intensive educational events, usually on weekends and are a combination of lectures, demonstrations, and practical sessions in the skills laboratory. Basic laparoscopic skills are typically required in order to participate. The laboratory session usually involves cadavers and animal stations are primarily used to introduce the participant to new procedure-specific instrumentation. The majority of short courses focus on laparoscopic colectomy. Courses on laparoscopic rectal resection are rare and reserved for participants who are well versed in laparoscopic colectomy. Participants of short courses were found to increase the number of course-specific procedures that they performed following the course [71]. In addition, they were found to consistently overestimate their performance, as measured by a global rating scale, which raises an issue of adequate credentialing [72, 73].

Preceptorship

This type of training is based on one-to-one supervision of a less experienced surgeon by an expert, who acts as a preceptor. Frequently, inexperienced surgeons in a surgical group are coached by an experienced member of the group (in-house preceptorship) [74]. The supervision period can vary from several cases to several months, depending on the trainee level. It is a very practical method of training. Occasionally, the trainee spends a designated time at the teacher's institution (out-of-house preceptorship, mini-sabbatical). This method allows the trainee to participate at an institution with a higher volume of cases under the supervision of a busy preceptor, though difficulties can arise in obtaining the necessary hospital/state privileges. In addition, there are potential problems associated with working in an unfamiliar operating theatre, patient population, and/or language. This form of training allows the preceptor to intervene if the situation arises and also allows for direct feedback and constructive criticism. In difficult operations, the preceptor is also on hand to perform the more challenging parts of the procedure [75].

Supervision and Feedback

According to Gagne, an essential component of the external conditions for learning motor skills is the provision of feedback as close to the time of performance as possible [76]. This feedback and constructive criticism are only possible by mentoring and close supervision, both of which impact the trainee's performance. In fact, intra-operative instruction has been found to decrease the rate of errors in a randomized laparoscopic suture study [5]. Additionally, in a meta-analysis of outcomes of 6064 patients, Miskovic et al. found that trainees with an appropriate level of supervision generated the same complication, conversion, and mortality rates as expert laparoscopic colorectal surgeons. This is extremely important in the context of the modern world where patient safety is paramount. In the same study, the authors compared the outcomes of non-mentored and mentored trainees and found that the experienced trainer can further aid in intra-operative decision-making and the comprehension of anatomy [62]. Case selection for training purposes is also indirectly related to supervision, with laparoscopic sigmoid resection being the easiest [77]. Similarly, appropriate patient selection for training purposes revealed that male sex, past surgical history, obesity, high ASA class, and colorectal fistulae were associated with higher conversion rates [62].

Highly Structured Training Programmes

Reznick and MacRae observed that volume alone does not account for the skill level among practitioners and that deliberate practice is a critical process in the development of mastery and expertise [10]. In the clinical setting, this deliberate practice is best accomplished within the context of a structured and supervised training programme. Many countries have introduced more or less structured curricula for the training of advanced laparoscopic procedures. A primary example of this is the National Training Programme for laparoscopic colonic surgery (NTP, Lapco), which began in 2007 and was funded by the Department of Health for England to provide training for consultants who had not been trained in laparoscopic colorectal surgery. It was a highly transparent, integrated, and structured training programme focused on hands-on training in the operating room, with the consultant in training (trainee) closely supervised and mentored by an experienced laparoscopic colorectal specialist. The NTP also includes laboratory, enhanced recovery, and theatre team training courses, as well as the train-the-trainer courses for faculty (trainers) [78]. The structure involves candidate selection, cadaveric and animal courses, "in-reach" (training centre) and "out-reach" (trainee's own hospital) supervised operating, for sign-off procedures, and an audit process. Both the trainee and the trainer are obligated to complete the GAS (Global Assessment Score), both of which are submitted electronically to the central Lapco office. Results of this programme have estimated that proficiency could be accomplished within 20–30 cases. At the end of the programme, two unedited videos are required for successful sign off at the end of the training. Mackenzie et al. observed that supervised fellowship of this type is safe and provides training without compromising patient safety, as it reduces learning curve as compared to self-taught surgeons [61].

Practical Training Considerations

It is important to realize that the set of teaching skills used in laparoscopic colorectal surgery training is unique and varies not only among different surgical centres, but also among different trainers from the same teaching programme. Therefore, while it is possible to have a certain level of standardization in the teaching technique during the simulation phase of laparoscopic skills, and during animal or cadaver training (if available), the framework of the teaching techniques of the trainer should also be standardized, as was seen in the National Training Programme (Lapco).

It is expected that the trainer will address and introduce the following basic principles before teaching the new laparoscopic colorectal procedures:

1. The aim is to produce a safe and competent colorectal surgeon who is comfortable with the use of laparoscopy but who uses sound judgment in performing open procedures when necessary.
2. The trainee possesses basic, fundamental laparoscopic skills, including basic laparoscopic ambidexterity.
3. The trainee has been given a thorough explanation of the technique and understands what can be accomplished at each particular stage of the procedure.
4. The trainee has been informed of, and understands, all necessary safety measures.
5. The trainee has been made aware of appropriate patient selection and how a thorough pre-operative workup should be conducted.
6. The trainee is aware how adequate laparoscopic exposure of the operating field is achieved.
7. The trainee has been instructed on and understands the macro-retraction and micro-retraction concept (see below).
8. The trainee is aware that there is a stepwise approach to each procedure.
9. The trainee is aware of the benefits of video recording of the laparoscopic phase and thorough video analysis following the procedure.
10. The trainee has been introduced to different approaches for each procedure.

Further elaboration of these principles and how the training protocol should be structured to address them are described below.

The Safe and Competent Laparoscopic Colorectal Surgeon

It is very important to remember that laparoscopy is a beneficial tool for the right patient in the right situation. With this in mind, it should be emphasized that utilization of open surgery when laparoscopy becomes too difficult is a sign of good judgment and maturity of the surgeon, and not an indication of failure [79].

Basic, Fundamental Laparoscopic Skills

Each trainee beginning the laparoscopic colorectal surgery training program should possess basic fundamental laparoscopic skills. These are most often obtained in the simulation laboratory and by performing procedures such as laparoscopic cholecystectomy and laparoscopic appendectomy. In addition, experience obtained from laparoscopic ventral hernia repair or laparoscopic adhesiolysis exposes the trainee to multiple quadrants of the abdominal cavity. These procedures also enable the trainee to become familiar with the concept of dynamic retraction and to learn how to quickly adjust to a changing anatomical environment, something that is more common in laparoscopic colorectal surgery due to the omnipresence of the small bowel and redundancy and tortuosity of the colon. This is also relevant to the significant variability of both colonic flexures and the sigmoid colon. Difficulty in acquiring the skill of bimanual dexterity (ambidexterity) is well documented in the literature [36, 80]. This skill is necessary in laparoscopic colorectal surgery and verbal feedback and demonstration are necessary in the process of improving this skill [81].

Understanding the Procedure

In the first cases of laparoscopic colon surgery, the trainee is typically preoccupied with adjusting to the new environment (hardware, setup, unfamiliar team, different view of the anatomy). It is therefore imperative to perform a simple and easy to remember role assignment, explaining what task the trainee will perform at each phase of the procedure. In most instances, laparoscopic mobilization of the colon can be achieved by using three working instruments and one camera, in a procedure performed by two surgeons. This translates into an easy to understand role assignment for the trainer, the assistant and the trainee.

It is very common that the main surgeon controls the conduct of the operation by operating the camera and providing retraction (passive role). Thus, the role of the trainee is to perform dissection (active role), either blunt or sharp, and or to help with retraction. Because this concept is very similar to teaching open surgery, it is often perceived that the trainee has performed the procedure when, in fact, the main surgeon has remained in control and orchestrated the entire procedure. This is a very important concept that allows the trainee to build confidence while performing laparoscopic colon procedures by encouraging them to be active assistants if they are not already performing the case.

Mobilization of either the left or right side of the colon always consists of two phases of dissection in the lower and upper quadrants. Before each procedure, the trainee should become familiar with the hand, instrument, and task assignment for each of the parts of the procedure, and regularly review these role assignments. Again, it is important for the trainee to possess sufficient ambidextrous skills.

Laparoscopic colon mobilization can be achieved using several approaches. The trainee should be taught what is expected with each procedure in the majority of patients. This includes the boundaries of what can and cannot be accomplished safely using the laparoscopic technique, and includes identifying unfavourable anatomy. The trainee should also understand the amount of colonic mobilization in each part of the procedure, as well as when to change the approach to another quadrant. Special emphasis should be placed on when to convert the procedure to the extracorporeal phase, and what can be accomplished during this phase. The extracorporeal phase is often as important as the laparoscopic phase, though it accounts for only a fraction of the entire procedure.

Within basic laparoscopic colorectal surgery training, it is not always possible to teach the beginner how to perform all steps of a colectomy during the laparoscopic phase. Some of the final steps can be accomplished more safely and quickly during the extracorporeal phase, *e.g.* vessel or bowel control. Defining those steps depends on the patient body habitus, complexity of the case, and the surgeon's experience. During basic training the trainee will often have only the experience of 20 to 30 colectomy cases before finishing the programme and subsequently attempting to perform those procedures independently. It is also important to teach what can be safely and efficiently performed during the extracorporeal phases. The same amount of experience achieved during the postgraduate period, within the context of the structured fellowship, is believed to be more effective and can often incorporate rectal dissection.

Necessary Safety Measures

The trainee should be made aware of all necessary safety measures. These include proper patient positioning on the operating table, prevention of sliding off the table, achieving appropriate steep tilt of the operating table, ensuring adequate padding of joints and bony prominences (to prevent pressure sores and peripheral neuropathy), obtaining safe abdominal access to establish pneumoperitoneum, and safely introducing instruments once the patient is in the tilted position (instruments should be directed towards the anterior abdominal wall to prevent small bowel injury).

Special attention should also be given to safety during the dissection. If a monopolar cautery hook is used, dissection should be performed layer by layer, always visualizing the tissue to be cauterized. If bipolar cautery, radiofrequency or ultrasonic clamping and cutting devices are used, special caution and appropriate exposure should be provided in order to avoid injury to the bowel, ureter, nerve, or vascular structures (marginal colic artery). If an inadvertent bowel injury occurs, most often serosal tears, the trainee should know how to repair simple bowel injuries laparoscopically using a one or two layer suture technique. Finally, special attention should be given to blood vessel control, particularly when ligating the major mesenteric pedicles. All trainees should be well versed and comfortable with all energy sources to be used during the procedure. If the first hemostatic device fails, an automatic rescue plan must be implemented, either by a repeated attempt with the same device, pressure application, control of the squirting pedicle with a clamp or an Endoloop® or another device. If this also fails there should be rapid conversion to a hand-assisted or open procedure.

During the early training phase of laparoscopic colon surgery, the trainer is often in charge of the camera and in full control of the operating field, despite the fact that most of the dissection is performed by the trainee. Continual verbal cues by the trainer should provide sufficient guidance as to how and where to perform retraction or dissection. Explanation of the embryologic layers and identifying the correct tissue plane is often necessary.

Patient Selection and Pre-operative Workup

Although it is not always possible to select the best patient for every teaching case, it should be defined which patients are ideally suited for teaching laparoscopic colorectal surgery. Miskovic et al. as mentioned above, studied this issue [59]. In the authors' opinion, medium to tall patients with a BMI of 20–26 are likely to have favourable and standard anatomy. Patients with very low BMI (<20) and shorter statue may create a challenge due to thin embryologic layers that are not separated by adipose tissue. This can result in loss of the correct tissue plane resulting in a defect in the mesentery and oozing from the mesenteric vessels. In addition, the small bowel mesentery in very short individuals is difficult to retract and can obscure the operating field. Likewise, in patients with a high BMI (>27) it can be too difficult to expose the colonic mesenteric root. Small bowel obscuring the operating field can be a significant problem. Additional challenges occur when performing vascular pedicle control and during the transection of thick mesentery. Because the part of the colon being dissected is often heavy, its mesentery is prone to fracture during retraction, which can result in mesenteric oozing. Exteriorization or extraction of the specimen will often require a larger than usual incision.

After patient selection, it is critical to complete a thorough pre-operative workup. A significant amount of information can be obtained in advance from the CT scans, which in many cases, have already been performed for oncologic reasons. With information to hand, a reasonable decision about approaching very large tumors laparoscopically can be made. Anatomy of the abdominal cavity should also be studied pre-operatively with the trainee if a CT scan is available.

Operating Field Exposure

In order to perform the procedure successfully and to provide the best possible learning experience, the operating field should be optimally exposed. This is normally accomplished by a steep tilt of the operating table, allowing the small bowel to drop out of view field by gravity. A common problem during the initial phase of a surgeon's laparoscopic colorectal experience is insufficient tilt of the table, often due to reluctance of the anaesthetist. Thus, recognizing how much tilt can be applied safely is important and can be determined before draping the patient. It should be noted that prolonged tilt can lead to peripheral neuropathy [82].

Another common mistake seen with an inexperienced trainee is a struggle to obtain proper exposure. This can be easily solved by adding one or two extra ports and involving an assistant. Because laparoscopic colorectal procedures are performed over multiple quadrants of the abdominal cavity, it can be easy to lose the proper horizontal camera orientation [6]. Therefore, it can be helpful from time to time to view the entire operative field. This helps not only the person controlling the camera but also the trainee to conceptualize the operating field and adjust the position, as well as the instruments, as needed. The trainer should also keep in mind that inexperienced surgeons are more likely to injure tissue inadvertently during retraction, particularly when the retracting instruments are located beyond the field of view [35]. For this reason, the trainee should be instructed not to grab the bowel while retracting, but to instead gently push on the mesentery or the bowel itself. A useful exercise for teaching the trainee how to gently handle the bowel is to perform "running the bowel" during selected cases.

Once the initial operating field is exposed, it is imperative to maintain it in clean and proper embryologic layers for the entire case. Bloodless conduct of the operation is crucial, especially during teaching cases and the trainer should point out the appropriate embryologic layers. Gas dissection is often helpful and typically occurs once dissection is performed in the proper layer. This is often initiated by incision with a monopolar cautery. Subsequent dissection can be then performed bluntly if a bloodless plane is identified or with the use of monopolar cautery, if appropriate retraction is applied. It is important to remember that Toldt's fascia is comprised of several layers of thinner fasciae and dissection can be carried out between any of these layers. The deeper layers contain small squiggly vessels that can be disrupted if dissection is performed too deeply, resulting in bleeding and obscured planes of dissection. Since it is more likely that deeper layers of Toldt's fascia will be entered during the medial to lateral approach, care should be taken to identify the most superficial layer of Toldt's fascia at the beginning of the retroperitoneal dissection, which should be left in situ.

Macroretraction and Microretraction

It is important for the trainee to understand the concept of macro-retraction and micro-retraction. The term "macro-retraction" refers to retraction of a large organ such as the colon, bladder or omentum. This is often achieved using a laparoscopic grasper. The structure is usually grasped, moved, and held in a position that will allow for finer dissection in the focused field. The grasper is typically kept beyond the operative field and care must be taken to avoid injuring the retracted organ. The term "micro-retraction" refers to providing the necessary tissue tension in the area where finer dissection is performed. This dissection is performed in the field of view and any instrument can provide the retraction. The trainee must be ambidextrous enough to be able to provide both types of retraction with either hand.

Stepwise Approach

A stepwise approach to surgical training has been incorporated into many specialties, including laparoscopic colectomy training, where each procedure is broken down into simpler steps. Trainees are required to perform the same step in each procedure until they have demonstrated proficiency, at which point they advance to the next planned step. This approach allows for a safe and timely progression of the operation, as well as evaluation of the trainee and documentation of the learning curve. Often, the individual steps can be grouped into the larger steps, allowing the fast-learning trainees to become proficient more quickly. The proficiency-gain of each resident should be considered on a case-by-case basis.

Video Recording and Analysis

It is always surprising to see how many details of the operation can be noticed during the video review process that were not seen during the operation. This can often include proper camera positioning to allow both surgeons to orient themselves in the multi-quadrant abdominal field. Other elements include identification of proper tissue planes (retroperitoneal dissection), synchrony and coordination of movement. It is believed that simple video analysis sensitizes the trainee to keep the operating field clear, both by bloodless dissection and proper orientation. This leads to important habits acquired by the trainee, which then allows for clean and anatomical surgery to be performed in the future.

Learning Various Approaches

It is important for the trainee to become familiar with alternative approaches in laparoscopic colorectal surgery. Though one approach can be used in the majority of cases, this is not always the case. For example, while some surgeons prefer the inferior to superior approach for laparoscopic right colectomy, it may not be possible to do so safely if there is a large caecal tumor. Likewise, the medial to lateral approach may not be appropriate when large lymph nodes are found surrounding the ileocolic pedicle. This same medial to lateral approach during left colectomy may also not be possible in very obese individuals, in whom visualisation of the root of the colonic mesentery may be impossible. In these cases, the alternative option of choice would be the lateral to medial approach, which may avoid conversion to open surgery. Once familiar with the alternative approaches, the trainee maintains the necessary skills by periodically using them.

Summary

Teaching the advanced laparoscopic skills needed for colorectal procedures requires a different approach to that used to teach open surgery. Mastering basic laparoscopic skills is a 'sine qua non' before advanced training begins. The proficiency-gain curve in laparoscopic colorectal surgery is prolonged and can be shortened by adequate supervision and mentoring of the trainee. Incorporation of the training into the structured curriculum allows for acquisition of the necessary skills without compromising patient safety.

References

1. Halsted WS. The training of the surgeon. Bull Johns Hopkins Hosp. 1904;15:267–76.
2. Bergamaschi R. Farewell to "see one, do one, teach one"? Editorial Surg Endosc. 2001;15:637.
3. Figert PL, Park AE, Witzke DB, Schwartz RW. Transfer of training in acquiring laparoscopic skills. J Am Coll Surg. 2001;193(5):533–7.
4. Gallagher AG, Al-Akash M, Seymour NE, Satava RM. An ergonomic analysis of the effects of camera rotation on laparoscopic performance. Surg Endosc. 2009;23(12):2684–91.
5. Bergamaschi R, Dicko A. Instruction versus passive observation: a randomized educational research study on laparoscopic suture skills. Surg Laparosc Endosc Percutan Tech. 2000;10(5):319–22.
6. Uchal M, Haughn C, Raftopoulos Y, Hussain F, Reed JF, Tjugum J, Bergamaschi R. Robotic camera holder as good as expert camera holder: a randomized crossover trial. Surg Laparosc Endosc Percutan Tech. 2009;19(3):272–5.
7. Arora S, Sevdalis N, Aggarwal R, Sirimanna P, Darzi A, Kneebone R. Stress impairs psychomotor performance in novice laparoscopic surgeons. Surg Endosc. 2010;24(10):2588–93. Epub 2010 Mar 31.
8. Haluck RS, Krummel TM. Computers and virtual reality for surgical education in the 21st century. Arch Surg. 2000;135(7):786–92.
9. Schmidt RA. Processing information and making decisions. In: Motor learning and performance. Champain: Human Kinetics Publishing; 1991. p. 26–8.
10. Reznick RK, MacRae H. Teaching surgical skills–changes in the wind. N Engl J Med. 2006;355(25):2664–9.
11. Fitts PM, Posner MI. Human performance. Belmont: Brooks/Cole; 1967.
12. Kaufman HH, Wiegand RL, Tunick RH. Teaching surgeons to operate–principles of psychomotor skills training. Acta Neurochir (Wien). 1987;87(1–2):1–7. Review.
13. Aggarwal R, Darzi A, Grantcharov TP. A systematic review of skills transfer after surgical simulation training. Ann Surg. 2008;248(4):690–1; author reply 691.
14. Mahmood T, Darzi A. The learning curve for a colonoscopy simulator in the absence of any feedback: no feedback, no learning. Surg Endosc. 2004;18(8):1224–30.
15. Rogers DA, Regehr G, Howdieshell TR, Yeh KA, Palm E. The impact of external feedback on computer-assisted learning for surgical technical skill training. Am J Surg. 2000;179(4):341–3.
16. Xeroulis GJ, Park J, Moulton CA, Reznick RK, Leblanc V, Dubrowski A. Teaching suturing and knot-tying skills to medical students: a randomized controlled study comparing computer-based video instruction and (concurrent and summary) expert feedback. Surgery. 2007;141(4):442–9.
17. Uchal M, Tjugum J, Martinsen E, Qiu X, Bergamaschi R. The impact of sleep deprivation on product quality and procedure effectiveness in a laparoscopic physical simulator: a randomized controlled trial. Am J Surg. 2005;189(6):753–7.
18. Moulton CA, Dubrowski A, Macrae H, Graham B, Grober E, Reznick R. Teaching surgical skills: what kind of practice makes perfect?: a randomized, controlled trial. Ann Surg. 2006;244(3):400–9.
19. Barnes RW, Lang NP, Whiteside MF. Halstedian technique revisited. Innovations in teaching surgical skills. Ann Surg. 1989;210(1):118–21.

20. Rosser JC, Rosser LE, Savalgi RS. Skill acquisition and assessment for laparoscopic surgery. Arch Surg. 1997;132(2):200–4.
21. Uchal M, Raftopoulos Y, Tjugum J, Bergamaschi R. Validation of a six-task simulation model in minimally invasive surgery. Surg Endosc. 2005;19(1):109–16.
22. Jones MB, Kennedy RS. Isoperformance curves in applied psychology. Hum Factors. 1996;38(1):167–82.
23. Palter VN. Comprehensive training curricula for minimally invasive surgery. J Grad Med Educ. 2011;3(3):293–8.
24. Fried GM, Feldman LS, Vassiliou MC, Fraser SA, Stanbridge D, Ghitulescu G, Andrew CG. Proving the value of simulation in laparoscopic surgery. Ann Surg. 2004;240(3):518–25; discussion 525–8.
25. Vassiliou MC, Feldman LS, Andrew CG, Bergman S, Leffondré K, Stanbridge D, Fried GM. A global assessment tool for evaluation of intraoperative laparoscopic skills. Am J Surg. 2005;190(1):107–13.
26. Vassiliou MC, Ghitulescu GA, Feldman LS, Stanbridge D, Leffondré K, Sigman HH, Fried GM. The MISTELS program to measure technical skill in laparoscopic surgery: evidence for reliability. Surg Endosc. 2006;20(5):744–7.
27. Jordan JA, Gallagher AG, McGuigan J, McGlade K, McClure N. A comparison between randomly alternating imaging, normal laparoscopic imaging, and virtual reality training in laparoscopic psychomotor skill acquisition. Am J Surg. 2000;180(3):208–11.
28. Sroka G, Feldman LS, Vassiliou MC, Kaneva PA, Fayez R, Fried GM. Fundamentals of laparoscopic surgery simulator training to proficiency improves laparoscopic performance in the operating room-a randomized controlled trial. Am J Surg. 2010;199(1):115–20.
29. Datta V, Bann S, Aggarwal R, Mandalia M, Hance J, Darzi A. Technical skills examination for general surgical trainees. Br J Surg. 2006;93(9):1139–46.
30. Satava RM. Identification and reduction of surgical error using simulation. Minim Invasive Ther Allied Technol. 2005;14(4):257–61.
31. Grantcharov TP, Kristiansen VB, Bendix J, Bardram L, Rosenberg J, Funch-Jensen P. Randomized clinical trial of virtual reality simulation for laparoscopic skills training. Br J Surg. 2004;91(2):146–50.
32. Lee JY, Mucksavage P, Kerbl DC, Osann KE, Winfield HN, Kahol K, McDougall EM. Laparoscopic warm-up exercises improve performance of senior-level trainees during laparoscopic renal surgery. J Endourol. 2012;26(5):545–50.
33. Bridges M, Diamond DL. The financial impact of teaching surgical residents in the operating room. Am J Surg. 1999;177(1):28–32.
34. Aggarwal R, Ward J, Balasundaram I, Sains P, Athanasiou T, Darzi A. Proving the effectiveness of virtual reality simulation for training in laparoscopic surgery. Ann Surg. 2007;246(5):771–9.
35. Neary PC, Boyle E, Delaney CP, Senagore AJ, Keane FB, Gallagher AG. Construct validation of a novel hybrid virtual-reality simulator for training and assessing laparoscopic colectomy; results from the first course for experienced senior laparoscopic surgeons. Surg Endosc. 2008;22(10):2301–9.
36. LeBlanc F, Champagne BJ, Augestad KM, Neary PC, Senagore AJ, Ellis CN, Delaney CP, Colorectal Surgery Training Group. A comparison of human cadaver and augmented reality simulator models for straight laparoscopic colorectal skills acquisition training. J Am Coll Surg. 2010;211(2):250–5.
37. Essani R, Scriven RJ, McLarty AJ, Merriam LT, Ahn H, Bergamaschi R. Simulated laparoscopic sigmoidectomy training: responsiveness of surgery residents. Dis Colon Rectum. 2009;52(12):1956–61.
38. Cesanek P, Uchal M, Uranues S, Patruno J, Gogal C, Kimmel S, Bergamaschi R. Do hybrid simulator-generated metrics correlate with content-valid outcome measures? Surg Endosc. 2008;22(10):2178–83. Epub 2008 Jul 12.
39. Milsom JW, Böhm B, Decanini C, Fazio VW. Laparoscopic oncologic proctosigmoidectomy with low colorectal anastomosis in a cadaver model. Surg Endosc. 1994;8(9):1117–23.

40. Giger U, Frésard I, Häfliger A, Bergmann M, Krähenbühl L. Laparoscopic training on Thiel human cadavers: a model to teach advanced laparoscopic procedures. Surg Endosc. 2008;22(4):901–6. Epub 2007 Aug 18.
41. Ross HM, Simmang CL, Fleshman JW, Marcello PW. Adoption of laparoscopic colectomy: results and implications of ASCRS hands-on course participation. Surg Innov. 2008;15(3): 179–83.
42. Pattana-arun J, Udomsawaengsup S, Sahakitrungruang C, Tansatit T, Tantiphlachiva K, Rojanasakul A. The new laparoscopic proctocolectomy training (in soft cadaver). J Med Assoc Thai. 2005;88 Suppl 4:S65–9.
43. Sharma M, Horgan A. Comparison of fresh-frozen cadaver and high-fidelity virtual reality simulator as methods of laparoscopic training. World J Surg. 2012;36(8):1732–7.
44. Iordache F, Bucobo JC, Devlin D, You K, Bergamaschi R. Simulated training in colonoscopic stenting of colonic strictures: validation of a cadaver model. Colorectal Dis. 2015;17(7): 627–34. doi:10.1111/codi.12887.
45. Sturm LP, Windsor JA, Cosman PH, Cregan P, Hewett PJ, Maddern GJ. A systematic review of skills transfer after surgical simulation training. Ann Surg. 2008;248(2):166–79.
46. Zendejas B, Brydges R, Hamstra SJ, Cook DA. State of the evidence on simulation-based training for laparoscopic surgery: a systematic review. Ann Surg. 2013;257(4):586–93.
47. Palter VN, Grantcharov TP. Development and validation of a comprehensive curriculum to teach an advanced minimally invasive procedure: a randomized controlled trial. Ann Surg. 2012;256(1):25–32.
48. Buscaglia J, Karas J, Palladino N, Fakhoury J, Denoya P, Nagula S, Bucobo JC, Bishawi M, Bergamaschi R. Simulated transanal NOTES sigmoidectomy training improves the responsiveness of surgical endoscopists. Gastrointest Endosc. 2014. pii: S0016-5107(13)02700-4. doi:10.1016/j.gie.2013.12.017. Epub ahead of print.
49. Fox J, Gross CP, Longo W, Reddy V. Laparoscopic colectomy for the treatment of cancer has been widely adopted in the United States. Dis Colon Rectum. 2012;55(5):501–8.
50. Bardakcioglu O, Khan A, Aldridge C, Chen J. Growth of laparoscopic colectomy in the United States: analysis of regional and socioeconomic factors over time. Ann Surg. 2013;258(2):270–4.
51. Lucciarini P, Konigsrainer A, Eberl T, Margreiter R. Tumour inoculation during laparoscopic cholecystectomy. Lancet. 1993;342(8862):59.
52. Simunovic M, Baxter NN, Sutradhar R, Liu N, Cadeddu M, Urbach D. Uptake and patient outcomes of laparoscopic colon and rectal cancer surgery in a publicly funded system and following financial incentives. Ann Surg Oncol. 2013;20(12):3740–6.
53. Thompson BS, Coory MD, Lumley JW. National trends in the uptake of laparoscopic resection for colorectal cancer, 2000–2008. Med J Aust. 2011;194(9):443–7.
54. Cuschieri A. Nature of human error: implications for surgical practice. Ann Surg. 2006;244(5): 642–8. Review.
55. Dinçler S, Koller MT, Steurer J, Bachmann LM, Christen D, Buchmann P. Multidimensional analysis of learning curves in laparoscopic sigmoid resection: eight-year results. Dis Colon Rectum. 2003;46(10):1371–8; discussion 1378–9.
56. Bennett CL, Stryker SJ, Ferreira MR, Adams J, Beart Jr RW. The learning curve for laparoscopic colorectal surgery. Preliminary results from a prospective analysis of 1194 laparoscopic-assisted colectomies. Arch Surg. 1997;132(1):41–4; discussion 45.
57. Tekkis PP, Senagore AJ, Delaney CP, Fazio VW. Evaluation of the learning curve in laparoscopic colorectal surgery: comparison of right-sided and left-sided resections. Ann Surg. 2005;242(1):83–91.
58. Cima RR, Hassan I, Poola VP, Larson DW, Dozois EJ, Larson DR, O'Byrne MM, Huebner M. Failure of institutionally derived predictive models of conversion in laparoscopic colorectal surgery to predict conversion outcomes in an independent data set of 998 laparoscopic colorectal procedures. Ann Surg. 2010;251(4):652–8.

59. Miskovic D, Ni M, Wyles SM, Tekkis P, Hanna GB. Learning curve and case selection in laparoscopic colorectal surgery: systematic review and international multicenter analysis of 4852 cases. Dis Colon Rectum. 2012;55(12):1300–10.
60. Simons AJ, Anthone GJ, Ortega AE, Franklin M, Fleshman J, Geis WP, Beart Jr RW. Laparoscopic-assisted colectomy learning curve. Dis Colon Rectum. 1995;38(6):600–3.
61. Mackenzie H, Miskovic D, Ni M, Parvaiz A, Acheson AG, Jenkins JT, Griffith J, Coleman MG, Hanna GB. Clinical and educational proficiency gain of supervised laparoscopic colorectal surgical trainees. Surg Endosc. 2013;27(8):2704–11.
62. Miskovic D, Wyles SM, Ni M, Darzi AW, Hanna GB. Systematic review on mentoring and simulation in laparoscopic colorectal surgery. Ann Surg. 2010;252(6):943–51.
63. Martin JA, Regehr G, Reznick R, MacRae H, Murnaghan J, Hutchison C, Brown M. Objective structured assessment of technical skill (OSATS) for surgical residents. Br J Surg. 1997; 84(2):273–8.
64. Miskovic D. Proficiency gain and competency assessment in laparoscopic colorectal surgery – thesis (PhD). Imperial College London; 2012.
65. Miskovic D, Ni M, Wyles SM, Kennedy RH, Francis NK, Parvaiz A, Cunningham C, Rockall TA, Gudgeon AM, Coleman MG, Hanna GB, National Training Programme in Laparoscopic Colorectal Surgery in England. Is competency assessment at the specialist level achievable? A study for the national training programme in laparoscopic colorectal surgery in England. Ann Surg. 2013;257(3):476–82.
66. Kuhry E, Bonjer HJ, Haglind E, Hop WC, Veldkamp R, Cuesta MA, Jeekel J, Påhlman L, Morino M, Lacy A, Delgado S, COLOR Study Group. Impact of hospital case volume on short-term outcome after laparoscopic operation for colonic cancer. Surg Endosc. 2005; 19(5):687–92.
67. Ericsson KA. The acquisition of expert performance: an introduction to some of the issues. In: Ericsson KA, editor. The road to excellence: the acquisition of expert performance in the arts and sciences, sports and games. Mahwah: Erlbaum Lawrence Associates; 1996. p. 1–50.
68. Hyman N, Borrazzo E, Trevisani G, Osler T, Shackford S. Credentialing for laparoscopic bowel operation: there is no substitute for knowing the outcomes. J Am Coll Surg. 2007;205(4):576–80. Epub 2007 Aug 23.
69. Miskovic D, Ni M, Wyles SM, Parvaiz A, Hanna GB. Observational clinical human reliability analysis (OCHRA) for competency assessment in laparoscopic colorectal surgery at the specialist level. Surg Endosc. 2012;26(3):796–803.
70. Schlachta CM, Mamazza J, Grégoire R, Burpee SE, Pace KT, Poulin EC. Predicting conversion in laparoscopic colorectal surgery. Fellowship training may be an advantage. Surg Endosc. 2003;17(8):1288–91.
71. Houck J, Kopietz CM, Shah BC, Goede MR, McBride CL, Oleynikov D. Impact of advanced laparoscopy courses on present surgical practice. JSLS. 2013;17(2):174–7.
72. Lewis T, Aggarwal R, Sugden C, Darzi A. The adoption of advanced surgical techniques: are surgical masterclasses enough? Am J Surg. 2012;204(1):110–4.
73. Sidhu RS, Vikis E, Cheifetz R, Phang T. Self-assessment during a 2-day laparoscopic colectomy course: can surgeons judge how well they are learning new skills? Am J Surg. 2006;191(5):677–81.
74. Chikkappa MG, Jagger S, Griffith JP, Ausobsky JR, Steward MA, Davies JB. In-house colorectal laparoscopic preceptorship: a model for changing a unit's practice safely and efficiently. Int J Colorectal Dis. 2009;24(7):771–6.
75. Pigazzi A, Anderson C, Mojica-Manosa P, Smith D, Hernandez K, Paz IB, Ellenhorn JD. Impact of a full-time preceptor on the institutional outcome of laparoscopic colectomy. Surg Endosc. 2008;22(3):635–9.
76. Gagne RM. The conditions of learning. 4th ed. Orlando: Holt, Rinehart and Winston; 1985.
77. Jamali FR, Soweid AM, Dimassi H, Bailey C, Leroy J, Marescaux J. Evaluating the degree of difficulty of laparoscopic colorectal surgery. Arch Surg. 2008;143(8):762–7; discussion 768.

78. Wyles SM, Miskovic D, Ni Z, Acheson AG, Maxwell-Armstrong C, Longman R, Cecil T, Coleman MG, Horgan AF, Hanna GB. Analysis of laboratory-based laparoscopic colorectal surgery workshops within the English National Training Programme. Surg Endosc. 2011; 25(5):1559–66.
79. Schlachta CM, Sorsdahl AK, Lefebvre KL, McCune ML, Jayaraman S. A model for longitudinal mentoring and telementoring of laparoscopic colon surgery. Surg Endosc. 2009;23(7): 1634–8. Epub 2008 Dec 6.
80. Gumbs AA, Hogle NJ, Fowler DL. Evaluation of resident laparoscopic performance using global operative assessment of laparoscopic skills. J Am Coll Surg. 2007;204(2):308–13. Epub 2006 Dec 27.
81. Porte MC, Xeroulis G, Reznick RK, Dubrowski A. Verbal feedback from an expert is more effective than self-accessed feedback about motion efficiency in learning new surgical skills. Am J Surg. 2007;193(1):105–10.
82. Velchuru VR, Domajnko B, DeSouza A, Marecik S, Prasad LM, Park JJ, Abcarian H. Obesity increases the risk of postoperative peripheral neuropathy after minimally invasive colon and rectal surgery. Dis Colon Rectum. 2014;57(2):187–93.

Chapter 7
Teaching Advanced Laparoscopic Skills in Surgery for Morbid Obesity

Alice Yi-Chien Tsai, Alan Osborne, and Richard Welbourn

Introduction

Obesity was once considered as an epidemic only in Western societies. However over the last two decades, the prevalence of obesity and metabolic syndrome has been rapidly rising in developing countries [1]. In 2008, an estimate of 205 million men and 297 million women worldwide were obese, and obesity has become a global health problem [2]. An adult is considered to be overweight with a Body Mass Index (BMI) of 25–29.9 and obese with a BMI of 30 or above. The prevalence of obesity in England has trebled in the last 25 years. In 2010, 26 % of adult and 17 % of boys and 15 % of girls (aged 2–15) were obese in the UK [3]. According to the Foresight report, 60 % of man, 50 % of women and 25 % of children are estimated to become obese by 2050 [4].

Obesity imposes a significant human burden of disease, mortality, social exclusion and poor quality of life. It is closely associated with type 2 diabetes, hypertension, coronary heart disease, hypercholesterolemia, asthma, sleep apnoea, osteoarthritis and poor health status [5]. Obesity has a substantial human cost by contributing to the onset of disease and premature mortality. It also has serious financial consequences for the health service and economy [6]. In England, the direct costs to the NHS for treating overweight, obesity and related disease had

A.Y.-C. Tsai, MB ChB, BSc, MRCS (✉)
Upper Gastrointestinal Surgery, Musgrove Park Hospital, Taunton, Somerset TAI 5DA, UK
e-mail: a.tsai@imperial.ac.uk

A. Osborne, FRCS, MMED
Department of Bariatric Surgery, North Bristol NHS Trust, Southmead Hospital, Southmead Road, Bristol BS10 5NB, UK
e-mail: alan.osborne@nbt.nhs.uk

R. Welbourn, MD, FRCS
Dept Upper GI and Bariatric Surgery, Musgrove Park Hospital, Taunton, Somerset TAI 5DA, UK
e-mail: Richard.Welbourn@tst.nhs.uk

N. Francis et al. (eds.), *Training in Minimal Access Surgery*,
DOI 10.1007/978-1-4471-6494-4_7

increased from £479.3 million in 1998 to £4.2 billion in 2007; the indirect costs, in other words, the costs arising from the impact of obesity on the society had increased from £2.6 billion to £15.8 billion [4].

Bariatric surgery has proven to be significantly more effective than conventional medical therapy for the treatment of severe obesity, including reduced cardiovascular morbidities, prevention of some cancers, better glycaemic control for patients with type 2 diabetes and improved quality of life [7, 8]. In particular, the long running Swedish Obese Subjects (SOS) Study has demonstrated favourable results for surgery with long-term weight loss and improvement in obesity-related disease, resulting in a mortality benefit compared to conventional therapy at more than 15 years [7]. In 2009, Picot conducted a literature review to assess the clinical effectiveness and cost-effectiveness of bariatric surgery confirming the benefits in moderately to severely obese patients compared to non-surgical interventions [9].

The first health economic report of obesity surgery in England by the independent Office of Health Economics in September 2010, estimated around 140,000 people qualified for bariatric surgery under National Institute for Health and Clinical Excellence (NICE) guidelines, while the number of surgeries performed was only 3607 in 2009-10. "Shedding the Pounds" further reported that if just 5 % of NICE-eligible patients were to receive bariatric surgery, the total net gain to the economy within 3 years would be £382 million [10].

In order to meet the increasing demand for bariatric surgery, more bariatric centres need to be established with the capacity to deliver standardised bariatric training. Bariatric surgery is a highly demanding and challenging surgical therapy, and a multi-disciplinary evaluation is vital to providing best patient care. Additional services include specialised nursing staff, dietitians, psychologists, and a medical team of surgeons, anaesthetists, critical care specialists, and psychiatrists. This chapter outlines the commonly practised bariatric procedures and provides recommendations on setting up a bariatric service to support good clinical care and surgical training.

Bariatric Operations and Surgical Technique

According to the current NICE guidelines, bariatric surgery is recommended as a treatment for adults if the BMI is at least 40 kg/m^2, or 35 kg/m^2 or more with a weight loss responsive disease (Table 7.1) [11]. It is considered as a first line treatment if the BMI is greater than 50 kg/m^2 rather than repeating failed prior

Table 7.1 Obesity: NICE guideline [11]

Bariatric Surgery is a treatment option if ALL of the following criteria are fulfilled:
BMI ≥ 40, or 35 ≤ BMI <40 with significant disease that could be improved by weight loss.
Failure to achieve or maintain adequate and clinically beneficial weight loss despite all appropriate non-surgical measures for at least 6 months.
The patient has been receiving or will receive intensive management in a specialist obesity service.
The patient is generally fit for anaesthesia and surgery.
The patient commits to long-term follow up.

interventions. The operations were originally designed as restrictive or mal-absorptive procedures, but are now understood to alter the signalling mechanisms controlling appetite, satiety and glycaemic control.

Roux-En-Y Gastric Bypass

Roux-en-Y gastric bypass (RYGB) is the most commonly performed bariatric operation in the UK and USA. The Roux-en-Y type of gastrointestinal anastomosis was first introduced in the nineteenth century by the Swiss surgeon, César Roux. Roux was the first Professor of External Pathology and Gynaecology at the University of Lausanne and was well recognised throughout Europe as a surgical innovator and educator. He published several articles on gastroenterostomy, which was mostly performed for gastric outlet obstruction at that time. The Y connection was documented in the publication in 1897 but was subsequently abandoned by surgeons due to the high rate of marginal ulcers and mortality [12]. In 1950, Dr Edward Mason and colleagues at the University of Iowa Hospitals and Clinics modified the Roux procedure into the current anti-obesity gastric bypass based on the weight loss observed among patients undergoing partial stomach removal for ulcers [13, 14]. In 1994, Dr. Alan Wittgrove reported the first five cases of laparoscopic approach [15]. This was achieved through 5 to 6 small abdominal incisions with an induced pneumoperitoneum. Studies comparing clinical outcomes of open and laparoscopic procedures have shown that laparoscopic gastric bypass is associated with lower overall postoperative complications and mortality, shorter length of stay, and lower hospital costs [16, 17].

The procedure consists of (1) creating a small gastric pouch of no more than 5–6 cm that is separated from the fundus. MacLean et al. described the formation of vertical gastric pouch, where a pouch on the lesser curvature was made adjacent to a 28 or 30 Fr bougie using a stapler that made two double rows of staples with an interval of free tissue in between to permit division. The staple line on the pouch side was oversewn and the gastric side was inverted [18, 19]. (2) Reconstructing the GI tract in which the jejunum, usually between 15 and 50 cm from the ligament of Treitz, is divided and rearranged into a Y- configuration. The "Roux limb" is the section from the gastrojejunostomy to jejunojejunostomy anastomosis, which enables the outflow of the food from the gastric pouch into the jejunum, bypassing the duodenum (Fig. 7.1). The gastrojejunostomy can be created by linear stapling, circular stapling or hand-sewn techniques [20]. When applying the circular stapling technique, the anvil of the stapler can be inserted transorally or transabdominally [21, 22]. The biliary limb is anastomosed to the alimentary limb to form the common channel where food mixes with the digestive enzymes. Lengthening of the Roux limb and biliary limb leads to shortening of the common limb. The biliary limb is commonly kept short in the existing literature, leaving the length of the Roux limb open to debate. Studies in the early 1990s demonstrated an increase in excess body weight loss in patients with extended Roux limb of around 100–150 cm, compared to 40–75 cm [23, 24]. Roux limb length equal or greater than 150 cm is performed in superobese patients (BMI>50 kg/m^2) with limited evidence [23–27]. Metabolic

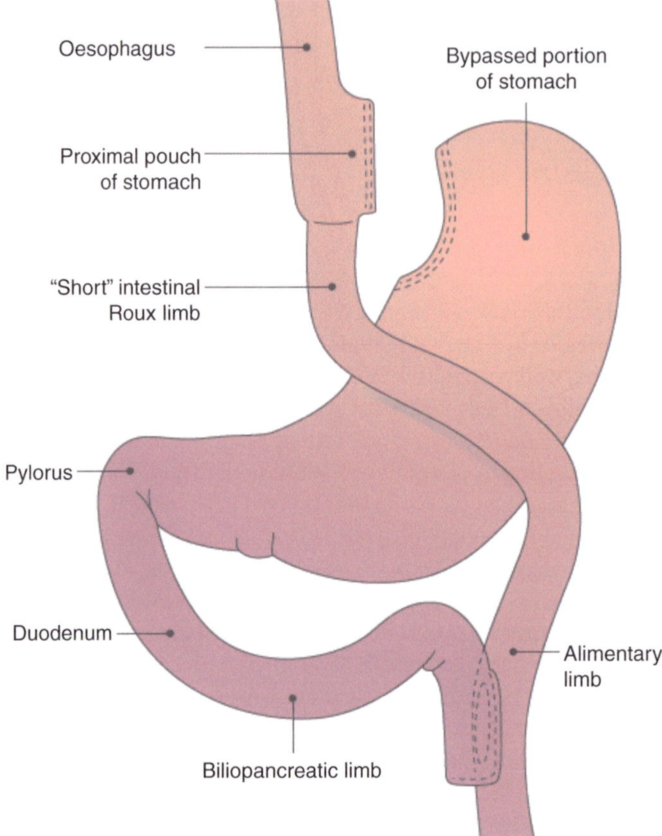

Fig. 7.1 Roux-en-Y gastric bypass (With permission from Elsevier [66])

complications and nutritional deficiency are likely to occur in patients with short common channels [23].

Studies have shown reduced hunger, increased satiety and altered bile salt concentrations in patients with RYGB, which are associated with exaggerated responses of anorexigenic intestinal hormones such as glucagon-like polypeptide-1 (GLP-1) and peptide YY (PYY); [26, 27] these changes in gut hormones are absent in gastric band surgery [28]. Changes in taste include food preferences with high-calorie foods becoming less appealing and less consumed. This was demonstrated using functional magnetic resonance imaging (MRI), which showed that activation of brain reward systems during evaluation of the appeal of high-calorie food was less after gastric bypass than gastric banding [29]. Energy expenditure also increases after surgery and research into mechanisms is ongoing.

Early post-operative complications include anastomotic leak, gastrointestinal bleed from the staple line, deep vein thrombosis, pulmonary embolism, and respiratory failures. Late complications include bowel obstruction, internal hernia, stomal stenosis, marginal ulcer, and vitamin/micronutrient deficiencies.

Gastric Banding

Belachew et al. first described the technique for laparoscopic adjustable gastric band (LAGB) in 1995 [30]. Since then, modified techniques and different types of gastric bands have been developed. The perigastric pathway was the traditional approach for tunnelling the band posteriorly. However, there was a tendency for the posterior wall of the stomach to prolapse through the band and therefore has been replaced by the pars flaccida approach [31]. A retrospective multicentre study compared the two approaches with more than 1200 patients in each treatment group. This showed a significantly higher rate of gastric pouch dilatation, intragastric migration and conversion to laparotomy in the perigastric group [32].

Five or six trocars are used, including one for the liver retractor. The dissection begins at the lesser curvature where an opening is made. Dissection continues through the retrogastric tunnel towards the angle of His. The band is introduced through a large trocar and placed at the top of the stomach, above the lesser sac, including the fat and vagus nerve branch within the band [33] (Fig. 7.2). The majority of surgeons achieve anterior fixation of the band by creating a gastro-gastric tunnel with interrupted sutures to reduce the risk of anterior slippage, however, the consequences on band erosion remain unknown. The access port for adjustment of band tightness is placed on the anterior rectus sheath and should be easily accessible for percutaneous needle puncture.

The primary mechanism of action of gastric banding is inducing a background of satiety and early post-prandial satiation. The feeling of satiety is likely to be mediated by the vagal receptors in the apex of the gastric cardia, and therefore the correct band placement is crucial to achieve the desired effect. Band adjustment is made with a non-coring deflected needle (Huber point needle). Follow up should be offered to patients every 4–6 weeks with the aim of achieving optimal restriction for individual patients. The Centre for Obesity Research and Education (CORE), Monash Medical School, Melbourne, Australia describes the optimal restriction as the "Green Zone" (Table 7.2), which is achieved by successive incremental adjustments and close monitoring of weight loss and symptoms. Patient follow-up plays an important role in the amount of excess weight loss (EWL); Shen et al. showed that patients who had more than six times of follow up within 1 year achieved 50 % EWL compared to the 42 % for those who had 6 or less follow up times (P=0005) [34].

LAGB has a low perioperative complication rate compared to RYGB. Late complications include band prolapse (slippage), band erosion, and access port infection. The clinical presentation of band prolapse can be non-specific and therefore difficult to diagnose. Symptoms include acid reflux, heartburn, coughing, choking spells and wheezing. Prolapse of the posterior wall of the stomach is managed by removal of the band and replacement of a new band via the pars flaccida pathway, whereas prolapse of the anterior wall can be managed by mobilisation and reduction of prolapse if the stomach is not overly oedematous [35].

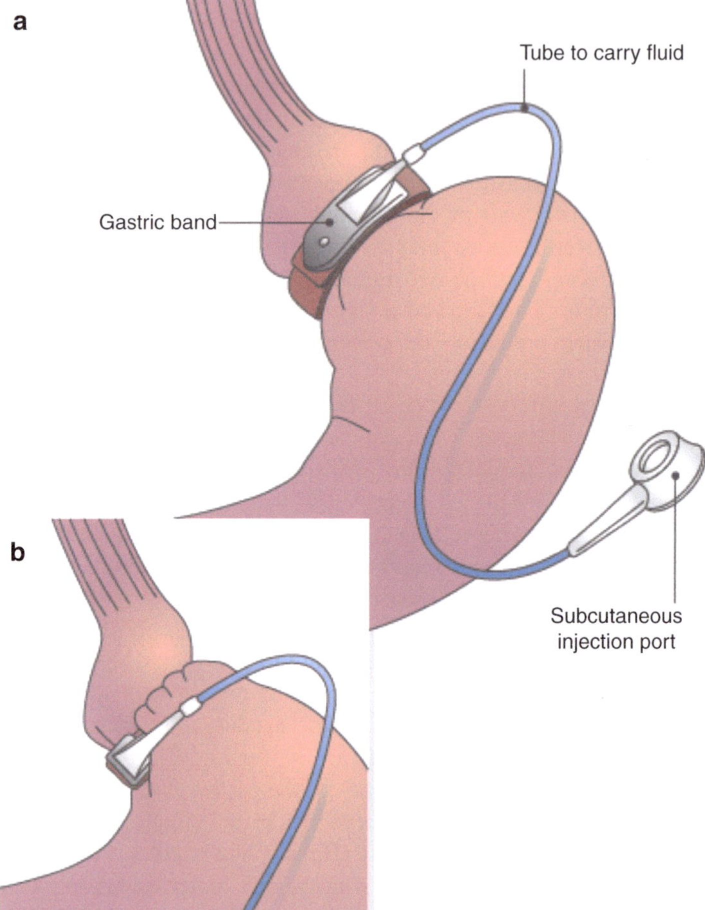

Fig. 7.2 (**a**) Gastric band with subcutaneous injection port, (**b**) Gastric band after filling [66]

Table 7.2 The Centre of Obesity Research and Education (CORE), Monash Medical School, Melbourne, Australia describes the "Green Zone" as the optimal adjustment for gastric band

Under filled	Green zone	Over filled
Hungry	Satiety	Dysphagia
Big meals	Small meals	Reflux/cough/regurgitation
Looking for food	Satisfy	Maladaptive eating.

Sleeve Gastrectomy

The first open sleeve gastrectomy was performed by Dr Doug Hess, Bowling Green, Ohio in 1998 as a part of the biliopancreatic diversion and duodenal switch procedure (BPD-DS) [36]. In 2000, Michel Gagner first described laparoscopic

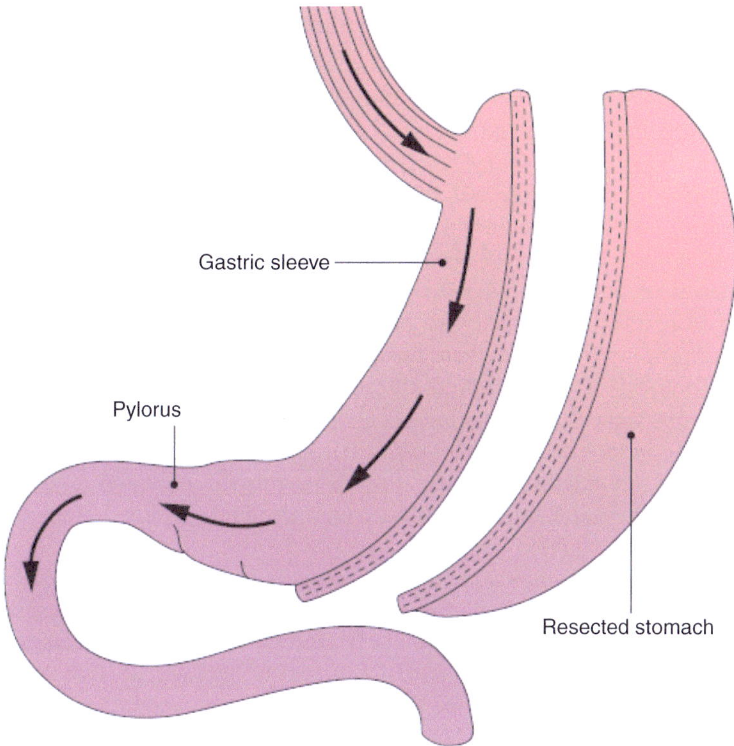

Fig. 7.3 Sleeve gastrectomy (With permission from Elsevier [66])

sleeve gastrectomy (LSG) as the first step of BPD-DS, which is now widely adopted [37, 38]. The greater omentum is divided with ultrasonic shears along the greater curvature up to the fundus and down to 2 cm proximal to pylorus. The angle of His is then dissected free from the left crus of the diaphragm. A 28–54 Fr bougie is inserted along the line of the lesser curvature to guide the dissection of creating a thin tube. The size of the gastric pouch is dependent on whether LSG was performed independently or as a part of BPD-DS [39]. The stomach is divided from the incisura angularis to the angle of His with the sequential use of linear stapling devices (Fig. 7.3).

Sleeve gastrectomy is now considered as an effective stand-alone procedure for high risk super-obese patients and is associated with improvement in comorbidities and a low complication rate [40, 41]. The mechanism of action is unclear, but it is thought to be mainly restrictive with some neurohumoral changes.

Complications of sleeve gastrectomy include staple-line bleeding, leak, and late stricture. Gastroesophageal reflux symptoms are common in the long term. A perceived benefit of the sleeve is that if there is weight regain afterwards, it is still possible to convert to another bariatric operation such as gastric bypass or duodenal switch.

Bilio-Pancreatic Diversion with Duodenal Switch

Professor Nicola Scopinaro first introduced the bilio-pancreatic diversion (BPD) in 1979 [42]. It was designed as a safer technique to the jejunoileal bypass performed from the 1950s to 1970s. It had significant nutritional and metabolic complications and therefore was modified to include a duodenal switch (DS) in an attempt to eliminate them [42]. BPD-DS is technically challenging and usually considered as a planned second stage or rescue operation (duodenoileostomy/ileo-ileostomy) after a sleeve gastrectomy. The gastrocolic ligament is divided from the distal antrum to proximal duodenum. The dissection of the duodenum ends at the point where the anterior pancreatic tissue joins the duodenal wall. A linear stapler is used to transect the duodenum. The common limb is measured 50–100 cm from the ileocaecal valve and the alimentary limb is therefore variable in length (about 200–300 cm). The ileum is divided at the point of measurement and the duodeno-ileostomy is performed as an end-to-end anastomosis with a circular stapler. The bilio-pancreatic limb is joined to the common limb by a side-to-side ileo-lieostomy.

The BPD-DS is a combination procedure that is both restrictive and malabsorptive. It produces effective weight loss in patients with a BMI > 50 and may be superior to RYGB in achieving weight loss [43]. Dorman and colleagues compared 190 patients who underwent primary BPD-DS between 2005 and 2010 to 139 RYGB patients. They found no difference between percent total weight loss between the two groups and significantly higher improvements in type 2 diabetes, hypertension and hyperlipidaemia in the BPD-DS group [44].

Patients having BPD-DS require rigorous life long medical and nutritional follow up as long-term nutritional and vitamin deficiencies occur at a significant rate [43].

Surgical Training in Bariatric Surgery

In the USA, the number of bariatric cases has grown from approximately 40,000 in 2000, to 80,000 in 2002 and to a current estimate of 113,000 cases per year [44, 45]. In the UK, there had been a 30-fold increase in the last decade to more than 8000 cases in 2011 [46]. Bariatric surgery is now possibly the commonest gastrointestinal operation in the USA and this has led to a significant increase in the number of bariatric programmes. A risk of this is that many surgeons might enter into bariatric practice without sufficient training and experience, or work in institutions without sufficient infrastructure to provide the necessary multidisciplinary structure for the overall care [47].

The current professional standards to accredit bariatric surgeons and institutes in the UK and USA are based on case volume, hospital infrastructure and staffing requirements for the multidisciplinary team [48, 49]. These requirements are established upon the strong evidence of improved patient outcomes under the care of high volume surgeons and high volume centres and the assumption that volume of cases directly reflects a surgeon's competency [50]. A bariatric training programme needs to meet the increasing clinical demand whilst maintaining patient safety.

Challenges in Bariatric Training

Two thirds of oesophago-gastric Upper Gastro-Intestinal trainees in the UK have shown a commitment towards training in Bariatric surgery (Fig. 7.4). However, trainees are not expected to attain full competence in advanced sub-speciality procedures by the time of their Certificate of Completion of Training (CCT) according to the Intercollegiate Surgical Curriculum Project (ISCP) surgical curriculum. The majority of trainees therefore feel unable to practise as a specialist at the end of their general surgical training (Fig. 7.5) [51]. As a result, almost 100 % of bariatric trainees wish to undertake a fellowship programme. A possible explanation is the apparent number of low volume bariatric units, suggesting less exposure to bariatric

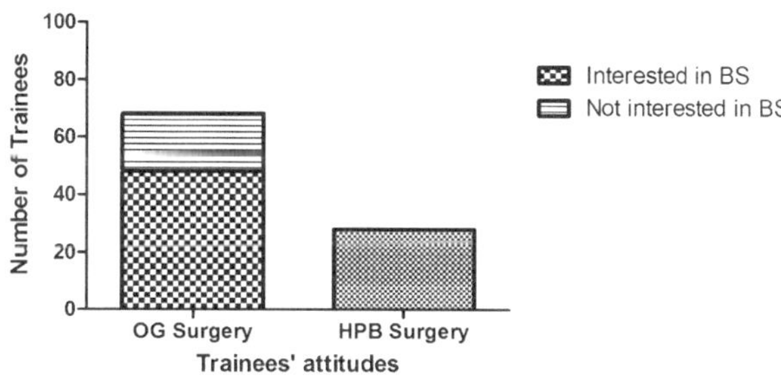

Fig. 7.4 Two thirds of OG trainees were interested in Bariatric surgery

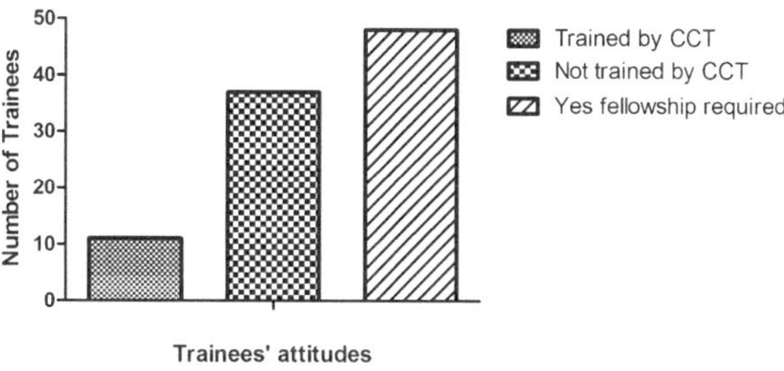

Fig. 7.5 The majority of trainees feel unable to practice as a specialist at the end of CCT

operations. Data from the UK suggests that only 20 bariatric surgeons operated on more than 100 procedures a year and only 11 hospitals carried out >200 procedures a year from 2008 to 2010 [18].

Proficiency-Gain Curve

The understanding of proficiency-gain curve forms the foundation of training development. A proficiency-gain curve is defined as the number of procedures that a surgeon needs to perform to reach a plateau in operating time, conversion rates, complications and mortality. Laparoscopic Roux-en-Y gastric bypass (LRYGB) is the most commonly performed operation and has received the most attention.

In 2002, Dr Oliak and colleagues analysed the first 225 consecutive LRYGB operations performed by one laparoscopic surgeon and showed that most of the reduction in operative time occurred over the first 75 patients [52]. The perioperative complication rate also decreased from 32 % for the first 75 patients to 15 % for the second 75 patients. A study done by Pournaras et al. in the UK similarly demonstrated a proficiency-gain curve of 100 in which the mean operative time decreased significantly after the first 100 patients [53]. Studies have shown that the early part of the proficiency-gain curve is associated with higher mortality and morbidity. A historical paper published by Flum & Dellinger in 2004 evaluated 30-day mortality of 3,328 patients who underwent obesity procedures over a 15-year study period. When the mortality was considered in a multivariable logistic regression analysis, only surgical inexperience and patients' comorbidities were associated with increased 30-day mortality [54]. The odds ratio of patient death within 30 days of hospital discharge was 4.7 times higher within the surgeon's first 19 procedures. One of the main objectives of bariatric surgery is to reduce mortality, and therefore the mortality of patients undergoing surgery should not be higher than patients without surgery. Adams et al. reported 7,925 RYGB performed by six surgeons between 1984 and 2002 in Salt Lake City, Utah; patients were matched for age, sex, and BMI . There was no difference in mortality between the operated (42 deaths) and non-operated (41 deaths) patients in the first year with a mortality of 0.52 % [55]. This implies that surgeons who perform elective RYGB should have an operative mortality of 0.5 % or less in the first year. The first UK National Bariatric Surgery Registry report to March 2010 showed a mortality rate of only 0.2 % for RYGB; complication rates varied from 1 to 22 % depending on the series. Any new surgeon must keep their outcomes within these parameters to avoid the proficiency-gain curve effect. Establishing evidence-based training methods is crucial in reducing the proficiency-gain curve, ensuring patient safety, minimising differences in complication rate and mortality during the proficiency-gain curve.

Educational Tools for Training and Education/Assessment

Courses and workshops have become increasingly common in the last 10 years to improve patient safety while surgeons are on the proficiency-gain curve. Options of obtaining training in LRYGB include 1–2 day courses, extended mentoring by an experienced surgeon, "mini-fellowships" which range from 1 to 6 weeks in duration, and 6–12 months fellowship [56]. The LRYGB can be broken down into its constituent parts, allowing task-based learning until each step is mastered. If trainees understand the steps of the procedure and become competent at individual tasks such as laparoscopic suturing then they start at a higher point on the proficiency-gain curve. Simulation and live animal models are commonly used in short courses; the animals are anaesthetised and provide in vivo conditions. This helps trainees master the procedure in a risk free environment and provides a good bridge to optimise time later spent with human cadavers. The bariatric training courses culminate in the cadaver course, which uses education theory on how we learn to optimise education outcomes. A relationship between the bariatric course and the experiential learning model can be seen in Fig. 7.6 [57]. Course participants move around the learning cycle starting with expert demonstrations and discussion of the surgery. This is followed by cadaveric dissection, reflection (self-assessed or formal by trainers) with "tips and tricks" to improve their performance and mentoring by expert faculty to modify surgical practice. Trainees then start around the cycle again with further surgery under guidance from the faculty. This optimises instruction in advanced laparoscopic techniques from the start of the operation. Details

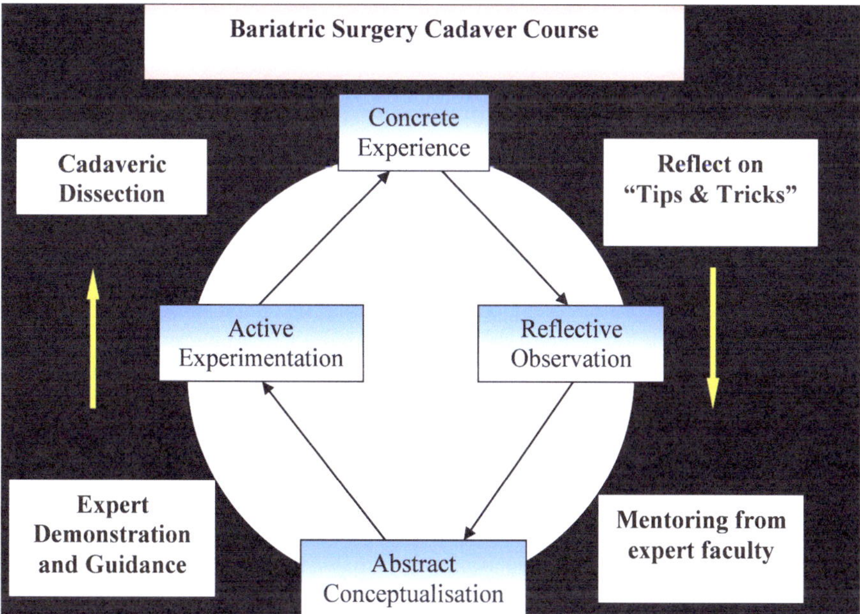

Fig. 7.6 A relationship between the Bariatric surgery cadaver course and the Experimental Learning Model (Adapted from Kolb, 1984 [53])

such as the operating theatre set-up, patient positioning, trocar placement and the efficient use of instrumentation are included. Non-technical skills such as teamwork leadership, safety and communication are also part of the operative training.

The bariatric training pathway cumulates in a fellowship of 6 months to 1 year depending on previous experience. Laparoscopic bariatric surgery requires mastery of a broad range of cognitive and technical skills. The curriculum of Bariatric and Metabolic Fellowship in the UK clearly states the requirement of fellows (Table 7.3) [58]. Fellowships are usually undertaken post-CCT or within the last 12 months of specialist training. Fellows are expected to achieve a minimum number of 100 weight loss operations of which >51 % are as the primary operating surgeon. A validated logbook including workplace based assessments (Table 7.4), in particular, procedure-based assessments (PBAs) are used as reflective templates in order to further reduce patient morbidity and mortality related to the proficiency-gain curve. The fellowship allows trainees to finish the proficiency-gain curve with a mentor and achieve competency as a bariatric specialist, including the opportunity to manage short and intermediate-term complications and be a part of the multidisciplinary bariatric team.

Learning and Teaching Style in Laparoscopic Bariatric Surgery

Learning styles have a great influence in operations with a long proficiency-gain curve like LRYGB. Although surgical trainees are more likely to adopt an activist or pragmatist learning style, a minority displays a strong preference for a reflector or theorist learning style. Therefore, surgeons teaching bariatric surgery have to consider the impact of varied learning styles and a uniform learning style cannot be assumed [59]. Acquiring a complex practical skill may be suited to an activist or pragmatist learning style. However, the theorist style is of benefit to understanding the underlying theory, knowledge and attributes required to practise bariatric surgery and the reflector learning style may facilitate trainees to practice the reflective observation part of the learning cycle (Fig. 7.7) [57].

Bariatric teaching must be able to accommodate all styles through balanced teaching and learning activities. If we consider LRYGB, reflectors/theorists will benefit most from thinking about the impending operation, reading up on the subject, discussing in advance and agreeing on a plan. They will complete the learning cycle by formally reflecting on the experience commonly using PBA (Fig. 7.8) [60]. Activists/pragmatists, on the other hand, will learn effectively from using models to learn the steps and then performing LRYGB under direct supervision. Due to the complexity of surgery, stronger activists may appreciate the opportunities of operating unsupervised and asking for help when needed. Stronger pragmatists may feel more comfortable to learn under supervision in a structured manner. The current bariatric training strategies are orientated around practical teaching, because the majority of surgical trainees fall in the activists/pragmatists groups. If the trainee is struggling to learn to perform LRYGB, or appears to have a proficiency-gain curve that is longer than normal, it is important to consider whether they have a reflector/theorist style. The teaching should be supplemented accordingly by increasing the focus on discussion of underlying principles of bariatric surgery and formalised reflection using the work-based assessment tools.

Table 7.3 Bariatric and Metabolic Fellowship Core Curriculum for the RCS National Surgical Fellowship Scheme [58]

Knowledge	
Epidemiology of obesity	
Pathophysiology of morbid obesity and the metabolic syndrome	
Therapeutic options for morbid obesity	
Indications for weight loss and metabolic surgery	
The principles of perioperative management of the obese patient	
Types of operations performed and mechanisms of action	
Complications of metabolic surgery and their management	
Revisional metabolic surgery	
Long term management of the bariatric patient following surgery	
Essential components of a bariatric service	
Psychology of the morbidly obese patient	
Clinical skills	
History and examination of the obese patient	
Interpretation of investigations in the obese patient	
Preoperative evaluation and optimisation	
Assessment of the post-operative bariatric patient	
Management decisions for early and late complications of bariatric surgery	
Technical skills	
Laparoscopic access in the morbidly obese	
Roux en Y gastric bypass	
Repair of internal hernia after gastric bypass	
Insertion of laparoscopic gastric band	
Aspiration of band port	
Emergency release of band for slippage	
Repositioning of band after slip	
Sleeve gastrectomy	
Participate in revisional surgery for obesity	
The management of general surgery in the super morbidly obese	
Professional attributes	
Participation and presentation of cases at bariatric MDT meetings	
Participation in departmental morbidity and mortality audit	
Knowledge of patient support group meetings	
Involvement in the debate and presentation of evidence-based surgery: Fellows are expected to participate in the Bariatric and Metabolic Trainees Collaborative.	
Involvement in surgical education with evidence of teaching and training: Fellows are expected to participate in the BOMSS annual training day.	
Target logbook (per 12 months)	
Total number of weight loss operations (primary surgeon in >51 %)	100
Minimum stapling/anastomotic operations	50
Minimum banding	10
Minimum revisional	5

Table 7.4 Workplace Based Assessments, Intercollegiate Surgical Curriculum Programme

Abbreviation	Full name	Content	Length of assessment	Lengnth of feedback
CBD	Case based discussion	Assessing how a clinical case is managed including considerations and reasons for actions.	15–20 mins	5 mins
CEX	Clinical evaluation exercise	Assessing clinical and professional skills through observations.	15–20 mins	5 mins
PBA	Procedure based assessment	Competencies and global assessment of performing a procedure/operation	Dependent on procedure	Dependent on procedure
DOPS	Direct observation of procedural skills in surgery	Assessing technical, operative and professional skills in basic diagnostic and interventional procedures of parts of procedures.	15–20 mins	5 mins
MSF	Multi source feedback	Peer assessment, by a range of co-workers including consultants,, junior doctors and other health care professionals.	N/A	N/A

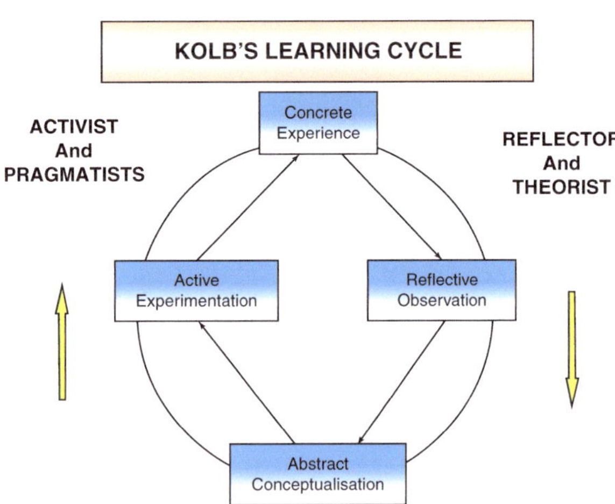

Fig. 7.7 A relationship between self-assessment and experiential learning model (Adapted from Kolb, 1984 [53])

Practical Application

Developing effective practical teaching is crucial and can be achieved by recording, and analysing operations performed by experts in the field. Laparoscopic recordings have been used as training aids to perform task analysis and motion analysis to optimise ergonomics and safety in bariatric procedures.

During a bariatric fellowship, trainees start by learning the skills required in laparoscopic gastric banding including access in obese patients, trocar placements,

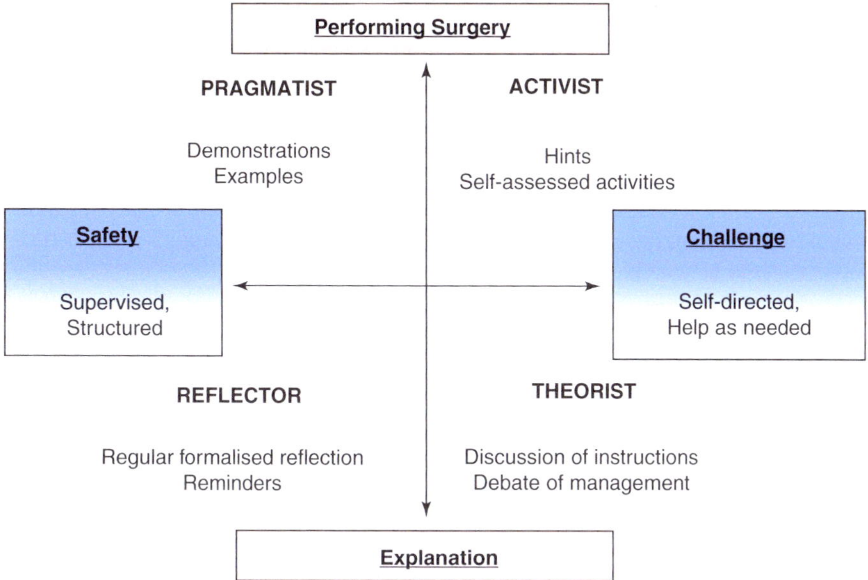

Fig. 7.8 A matrix for the application of SA PBA in the operating theatre (Adapted from Groat & Musson, 1996 [56])

liver retraction, pars flaccida approach and laparoscopic suturing. Some skills are transferrable from other major laparoscopic gastrointestinal surgical procedures.

Through evaluating videos of procedures performed by the authors and other experts, we divided LRYGB into two main parts – jejuno-jejunal anastomosis and gastro-jejunal anastomosis. We found that each part could be divided into a series of steps and performed with minimal variations, and therefore LRYGB is taught in a step-wise fashion. Trainees begin with learning jejuno-jejunal anastomosis by following the same sequence each time and practicing the task repetitively. They subsequently move on to learning gastro-jejunal anastomosis in the same manner. When the two parts are mastered, trainees then perform the entire operation in low risk patients and finally high-risk patients later along the proficiency-gain curve.

Video-enhanced feedback forms an integral part of continuing self-reflection and assessment. Trainees follow the trainer's guidance to reproduce the task and watch the video to refine economy of movements and review errors.

Future Directions – Competency Assessment in Bariatric Training

Surgical competency has been a hot topic of discussion in the UK in recent years along with the introduction of European Working Time Directive (EWTD) and reduced working time as a result. Studies have suggested that the reduction in working time has had a considerable negative effect on surgical training. The legal maximum working time is currently 48 h a week. In 2008, the Association for Surgeons in Training (ASiT) stated that to ensure optimal training with adequate time for exposure and high quality patient care with increased continuity of care, it would be necessary to return to a working week of approximately 65 h [61]. Due to the change in the working hours and pattern, surgical training changed from a time-based process into a competency-based one, where various aspects of a trainee's practice are formally validated by an objective assessment process [62].

Methods such as Objective Structured Assessments of Technical Skills (OSATS), Procedure-Based Assessments (PBAs) and Direct Observation of Practical Skills (DOPS) have been developed to improve and standardise the quality of the assessment process across the UK.

In addition to the shift to competency-based validation, surgical skills courses including simulations have also blossomed in response to the change as a result of EWTD. Bariatric surgery is a challenging specialty and the acquisition of psychomotor skills is essential. As the theatre time at work is reduced, surgical trainees need to seek exposure elsewhere within the bariatric training pathway without compromising patient safety and quality of care.

Establishing a Bariatric Service and Hospital Infrastructure

A bariatric programme is multi-disciplinary and requires substantial commitment from the surgeons and from the institution [63]. The team includes surgeons, nutritionists/dietitians, psychologists/psychiatrists, anaesthetists, critical care physicians, endocrinologists, respiratory physicians, and specialised nursing staff. Professional bodies including the International Federation for Surgery of Obesity and Metabolic Disorders, American Society for Bariatric Surgery, American College of Surgeons and British Obesity & Metabolic Surgery Society (BOMSS) have set up safety, quality, and excellence guidelines and accreditation schemes to ensure the best standards of patient care [47, 48].

The establishment of a bariatric surgery programme requires commitment and investment by the hospital/institution. It is important to create an obesity-friendly environment from the waiting area in an outpatient clinic to the operating theatre and post-operative recovery ward. The weight capacity of furniture including chairs, benches, examination couches and beds must be adequate to support the patient safely. Bariatric patients often require diagnostic investigations such as gastroscopy, upper GI contrast studies and CT scanning during the hospital stay or as an emergency. The bariatric surgeon should be familiar with the weight and size limit of the equipment at the hospital before putting patients through surgery as this may set an upper weight limit for patient selection. Some older hospital buildings were not structurally designed to cater for bariatric patients and therefore the load-bearing capacity of the floor and the fire-escape staircase and equipment should be assessed.

BOMSS published its professional standards for facilities performing bariatric surgery in March 2013, which are summarised below [48]:

Equipment and Safety

- *Weighing scales*: *readily available weighing scales that are accessible to obese patients both standing and seated.*
- *Outpatient clinics*: *chairs, wheelchairs, doorways and examination couches that have the requisite weight limits and are adequately sized.*
- *Wards*: *patients should be managed on designated wards equipped with items with suitable weight capacity/size including beds, pressure relieving mattresses, chairs, toilets, wheelchairs, commodes, hoists, zimmer frames, anti-embolism stockings, and bed spaces.*
- *Theatres*: *operating theatres should be equipped with suitable table, manual handling devices and anaesthetic equipment including transfer facilities, electric operating table, operating table extensions and footplates, difficult intubation equipment, onsite blood gas analysis, and readily available blood for transfusion. There must be an adequate supply of instruments available for emergency re-operation including a bariatric grade static retractor system for open surgery.*
- *Post-operative recovery and high dependency/intensive care*: *on-site level 2 critical care facilities certified to the Care Quality Commission standards are essential for units undertaking bariatric surgery other than straightforward gastric banding.*
- *Imaging*: *facilities should have availability or safe access to cross sectional imaging and fluoroscopic imaging of the upper GI track suitable for the majority of the patients.*

Staffing

- *Patients must have access to full range of specialist professionals in line with NICE guidelines including surgeons, bariatric physicians/endocrinologists, anaesthetists, nurses and dieticians.*
- *Resident Medical Officer must be supported by the availability of 24/7 consultant surgical and anesthetic cover.*

Staff Education

- *All surgeons need to commit to continuing medical education.*
- *Postoperative care pathways and escalation policies should be available for all staff and resident doctors.*
- *Appropriate sensitivity training should be offered to all hospital and clinical staff for bariatric patients*

Governance

- *Care pathways, escalation policies and protocols should be agreed.*

Follow Up and Audit

- *Facilities should be committed to long-term follow up of their patients with appropriate level of surgeon, dietician, psychology/psychiatric, GP and nursing input.*
- *Facilities should commit to long-term data collection with local and national audit of their results. Such audit data should be publically available.*

Summary and Centre of Excellence

Obesity is a serious public health issue in the Western world and rapidly climbing in developing countries. The data overwhelmingly suggest that bariatric surgery is currently more effective than conventional medical therapy including dieting and lifestyle interventions. As the bariatric practice is increasing worldwide, it is essential to safeguard the standard of bariatric training and facilities that provide bariatric services.

Laparoscopic bariatric surgery requires mastery of a broad range of cognitive and technical skills including the management of severely obese patients. In the UK, the bariatric training pathway cumulates in a fellowship of 6 months to 1 year, depending on previous experience. Structured training programmes adapt the teaching methods to the learning styles of trainees and facilitate trainees to go through the learning cycle under close supervision to minimise the proficiency-gain curve effect. Bariatric fellowships should be based in bariatric centres that can provide sufficient exposure, adequate volume and varieties of operations, and meet the professional standards in delivering patient centred multidisciplinary care.

Professional bodies award Centre of Excellence (CoE) in Metabolic and Bariatric Surgery designation to institutions and surgeons that meet the standard worldwide. In Europe, Middle East and Africa, standards are set by the International Federation for the Surgery of Obesity and metabolic disorders (IFSO) and the European Accreditation Council for Bariatric Surgery and Surgical Review Corporation. In the United States, the standard is set by the Metabolic Bariatric Surgery and Quality Improvement Program (MBSAQIP), a joint accreditation programme by the American College of Surgeons (ACS) and the American Society for Metabolic and Bariatric Surgery (ASMBS). CoE awards are thought to serve as the benchmark for patients, commissioners, and health insurers to ensure health care standards and outcomes.

However, a group at the University of Michigan Health System challenged the value of CoE in 2010 by publishing a study that showed accreditation of bariatric CoE did not predict the rate of serious complications for patients undergoing bariatric surgery [64]. In 2013, the two governmental insurance programme in the US, Medicare and Medicaid, proposed to remove the CoE requirement in commissioning bariatric facilities as the evidence was insufficient to demonstrate better outcomes in Bariatric CoE compared to non-accredited centres. Although the CoE accreditation is likely to continue to hold weight, this decision might jeopardise the standard of care and lead to a less regulated bariatric surgery market, quality of surgeons and training system [65].

References

1. Misra A, Khurana L. Obesity and the metabolic syndrome in developing countries. J Clin Endocrinol Metab. 2008;93:S9–30.
2. Finucane MM, Stevens GA, Cowan MJ, Danaei G, Lin JK, Paciorek CJ, et al. National, regional, and global trends in body-mass index since 1980: systematic analysis of health

examination surveys and epidemiological studies with 960 country-years and 9·1 million participants. Lancet. 2011;377:557–67.

3. Health Survey for England – 2010: Respiratory Health. The NHS Information Centre. 2011. Available from: www.ic.nhs.uk/pubs/hse10report.
4. Butland B, Jebb S, Kopelman P, McPherson K, Thomas S, Mardell J, et al. Foresight tackling obesities: future choices – project report. Foresight; 2007. Available from: www.foresight.gov.uk.
5. Mokdad AH, Ford ES, Bowman BA, Dietz WH, Vinicor F, Bales VS, et al. JAMA. 2003;289:76–9.
6. National Audit Office. Tackling Obesity in England. London: the stationery office; 2001. Available from: https://www.nao.org.uk/report/tackling-obesity-in-england/.
7. Sjöström L, Lindroos A, Peltonen M, Torgerson J, Bouchard C, Carlsson B, et al. Lifestyle, diabetes, and cardiovascular risk factors 10 years after bariatric surgery. N Engl J Med. 2004;351:2683–93.
8. Schauer PR, Kashyap SR, Wolski K, Brethauer SA, Kirwan JP, Pothier CE, et al. Bariatric surgery versus intensive medical therapy in obese patients with diabetes. N Engl J Med. 2012;366:1567–76.
9. Picot J, Jones J, Colquitt JL, Gospodarevskaya E, Loveman E, Baxter L, et al. The clinical effectiveness and cost-effectiveness of bariatric (weight loss) surgery for obesity: a systematic review and economic evaluation. Health Technol Assess. 2009;13(41):1–190.
10. Shedding the pounds. Obesity management, NICE guidance and bariatric surgery in England. Office of Health Economics; 2010. Available from: http://www.rcseng.ac.uk/news/docs/BariatricReport.pdf.
11. Obesity. Guidance on the prevention, identification, assessment and management of overweight and obesity in adults and children. NICE clinical guideline 43; 2006. Available from: http://www.nice.org.uk/guidance/index.jsp?action=download&o=30365.
12. Hutchison RL, Hutchison AL. Cesar Roux and his original 1893 Paper. Obes Surg. 2010;20:953–6.
13. Mason EE, Printen KJ, Blommers TJ, Lewis JW, Scott DH. Gastric bypass in morbid obesity. Am J Clin Nutr. 1980;33:395–405.
14. Story of Obesity Surgery [Internet]. American Society for Metabolic & Bariatric Surgery. [updated 2005 May 25, cited 2014 Jan 20]. Available from: http://asmbs.org/story-of-obesity-surgery/.
15. Wittgrove AC, Clark GW, Tremblay LJ. Laparoscopic gastric bypass, Roux-en-Y: preliminary report of five cases. Obes Surg. 1994;4:353–7.
16. Luján JA, Frutos MD, Hernández Q, et al. Laparoscopic versus open gastric bypass in the treatment of morbid obesity: a randomized prospective study. Ann Surg. 2004;239(4):433–7.
17. Nguyen NT, Goldman C, Rosenquist CJ, et al. Laparoscopic versus open gastric bypass: a randomized study of outcomes, quality of life, and costs. Ann Surg. 2001;234(3):279–89; discussion 289–91.
18. MacLean LD, Rhode BM, Nohr CW. Late outcome of isolated gastric bypass. Ann Surg. 2000;231:524–8.
19. MacLean LD, Rhode BM, Sampalis J, Forse RA. Results of the surgical treatment of obesity. Am J Surg. 1993;165:155–62.
20. Welbourn R, Fiennes A, Kinsman R, Walton P. The United Kingdom national bariatric surgery registry. First registry report to March 2010. Dendrite Clinical Systems; 2011.
21. De la Torre RA, Scott JS. Laparoscopic Roux-en-Y divided gastric bypass with transgastric anvil placement. In: Inabnet WB, Demaria EJ, Ikramuddin S, editors. Laparoscopic bariatric surgery. Philadelphia: Lippincott Williams & Wilkins; 2005. p. 116–22.
22. Kurian M, Roslin M. Laparoscopic Roux-en-Y gastric bypass: transoral technique. In: Inabnet WB, Demaria EJ, Ikramuddin S, editors. Laparoscopic bariatric surgery. Philadelphia: Lippincott Williams & Wilkins; 2005. p. 95–101.
23. Brolin RE, Kenler HA, Gorman JH, Cody RP. Long-limb gastric bypass in the superobese. A prospective randomized study. Ann Surg. 1992;215:387–95.
24. Bruder SJ, Freeman JB, Brazeau-Gravelle P. Lengthening of Roux-en-Y limb increases weight loss after gastric bypass: a prelimary report. Obes Surg. 1991;1:73–7.

25. Brolin RE. Long limb Roux en Y gastric bypass revisited. Surg Clin North Am. 2005;85: 807–17.
26. Christou NV, Look D, MacLean LD. Weight gain after short- and long-limb gastric bypass in patients followed for longer than 10 Years. Ann Surg. 2006;244:734–40.
27. Orci L, Chillcott M, Huber O. Short versus long Roux-limb length in Roux-en-Y gastric bypass surgery for the treatment of morbid and super obesity: a systematic review of the literature. Obes Surg. 2011;21:797–804.
28. Le Roux CW, Aylwin SJ, Batterham RL, Borg CM, Coyle F, Prasad V, et al. Gut hormone profiles following bariatric surgery favor an anorectic state, facilitate weight loss and improve metabolic parameters. Ann Surg. 2006;243:108–14.
29. Scholtz S, Miras AD, Chhina N, Prechtl CG, Sleeth ML, Daud NM, et al. Obese patients after gastric bypass surgery have lower brain-hedonic responses to food than after gastric banding. Gut. 2014;63(6):891–902. doi: 10.1136/gutjnl-2013-305008.
30. Belachew M, Legrand M, Vincenti VV, Deffechereux T, Jourdan JL, Monami B, et al. Laparoscopic placement of adjustable silicon gastric band in the treatment of morbid obesity: how to do it. Obes Surg. 1995;5:66–70.
31. O'Brien PE, Dixon JB, Laurie C, Anderson M. A prospective randomized trial of placement of the laparoscopic adjustable gastric band: comparison of the perigastric and pars flaccida pathways. Obes Surg. 2005;15:820–6.
32. Di Lorenzo N, Furbetta F, Favretti F, Segato G, De Luca M, Micheletto G, et al. Laparoscopic adjustable gastric banding via pars flaccida versus perigastric positioning: technique, complications and results in 2459 patients. Surg Endosc. 2010;24:1519–23.
33. Kini S, Rao R, editors. Review of obesity and bariatric surgery. Essential notes and multiple choice questions. New York: Informa Healthcare; 2012.
34. Shen R, Dugay G, Rajaram K, Cabrera L, Siegel N, Ren CJ. Impact of patient follow-up on weight loss after bariatric surgery. Obes Surg. 2004;14:514–9.
35. O'Brien P, Dixon JB. Laparoscopic adjustable gastric banding. In: Inabnet WB, Demaria EJ, Ikramuddin S, editors. Laparoscopic bariatric surgery. Philadelphia: Lippincott Williams & Wilkins; 2005. p. 75–84.
36. Hess DS, Hess DW. Biliopancreatic diversion with a duodenal switch. Obes Surg. 1998;8(3):267–82. doi:10.1381/096089298765554476.
37. De Csepel J, Burpee S, Jossart G, Andrei V, Murakami Y, Benavides S, et al. Laparoscopic biliopancreatic diversion with a duodenal switch for morbid obesity: a feasibility study in pigs. J Laparoendosc Adv Surg Tech A. 2001;11:79–83.
38. Milone L, Strong V, Gagner M. Laparoscopic sleeve gastrectomy is superior to endoscopic intragastric balloon as a first stage procedure for super-obese patients (BMI > or =50). Obes Surg. 2005;15:612–7.
39. Trelles N, Gagner M. Updated review of sleeve gastrectomy. Open Gastroenterol J. 2008;2:41–9.
40. Basso N, Casella G, Rizzello M, Abbatini F, Soricelli E, Alessandri G, et al. Laparoscopic sleeve gastrectomy as first stage or definitive intent in 300 consecutive cases. Surg Endosc. 2011;25:444–9.
41. Eisenberg D, Bellatorre A, Bellatorre N. Sleeve gastrectomy as a stand-alone bariatric operation for severe, morbid and super obesity. JSLS. 2013;17:63–7.
42. Scopinaro N, Gianetta E, Civalleri D, Bonalumi U, Bachi V. Biliopancreatic by-pass for obesity. II. Initial experience in man. Br J Surg. 1979;66(9):618–20.
43. Kelly J, Shikora S, Jones D, Hutter M, Robinson MK, Romanelli J, et al. Best practice updates for surgical care in weight loss surgery. Obesity. 2009;17:863–70.
44. Dorman RB, Rasmus NF, al-Haddad BJ, Serrot FJ, Slusarek BM, Sampson BK, et al. Benefits and complications of the duodenal switch/biliopancreatic diversion compared to the Roux-en-Y gastric bypass. Surgery. 2012;152:758–65.
45. Livingston ED. The incidence of bariatric surgery has plateaued in the U.S. Am J Surg. 2010;200:378–85.
46. Statistics on obesity, physical activity and diet: England, 2012. The NHS Information Centre; 2012. Available from: http://www.hscic.gov.uk/catalogue/PUB05131/obes-phys-acti-diet-eng-2012-rep.pdf

47. Melissas J. IFSO guideline for safety, quality and excellence in bariatric surgery. Obes Surg. 2008;18:497–500.
48. BOMSS Professional Standards Document March 2013. Available from: http://www.bomss.org.uk/pdf/clinical_services_standards/BOMSS-Professional-Standards-March-2013.pdf.
49. Resources for Optimal Care of Metabolic and Bariatric Surgery Patient 2014. Metabolic and Bariatric Surgery Accreditation and Quality Improvement Program. Available from: http://www.mbsaqip.info/?page_id=54.
50. Zevin B, Aggarwal R, Grantcharov TP. Volume-outcome association in bariatric surgery: a systemic review. Ann Surg. 2012;256:60–71.
51. Osborne A, Hammond J, Allum W. Manpower planning in upper GI surgery: right or wrong? J ASGBI. 2011;35:3–7.
52. Oliak D, Ballantyne GH, Weber P, Wasielewski A, Davies RJ, Schmidt HJ. Laparoscopic Roux-en-Y gastric bypass: defining the proficiency-gain curve. Surg Endosc. 2003;17:405–8.
53. Pournaras DJ, Jafferbhoy S, Titcomb DR, Humadi S, Edmond JR, Mahon D, et al. Three hundred laparoscopic Roux-en-Y gastric bypasses: managing the proficiency-gain curve in higher risk patients. Obes Surg. 2010;20:290–4.
54. Flum DR, Dellinger EP. Impact of gastric bypass operation on survival: a population-based analysis. J Am Coll Surg. 2004;199:543–51.
55. Adams TD, Gress RE, Smith SC, Halverson RC, Simper SC, Rosamond WD, et al. Long-term mortality after gastric bypass surgery. N Engl J Med. 2007;357:753–61.
56. Kothari SN, Boyd WC, Larson CA, Gustafson HL, Lambert PJ, Mathiason MA. Training of a minimally invasive bariatric surgeon: are laparoscopic fellowships the answer? Obes Surg. 2005;15:323–9.
57. Kolb DA. Experimental learning experience as a source of learning and development. London: Prentice Hall; 1984.
58. British Obesity & Metabolic Surgery Society. Bariatric and metabolic fellowship core curriculum for the RCS national surgical fellowship scheme. 2013. Available from: http://www.bomss.org.uk/pdf/Bariatric%20and%20Metabolic%20Fellowship%20Core%20Curriculum%20for%20Post-CCT%20Fellows.pdf.
59. Osborne AJ, Hawkins SC, James A, Pournaras D, Pullyblank A. Training in current medical education: surgeons are different from their medical colleagues. B Roy Coll Surg Engl. 2012;94:242–5.
60. Groat A, Musson T. Learning styles: individualising computer based learning environments. Assoc Learn Technol J. 1996;3:53–62.
61. Cresswell B, Marron C, Hawkins W, Harrison E, Fitzgerald, von Roon A. Optimising working hours to provide quality in training and patient safety. A position statement by the Association of Surgeons in Training. 2009.
62. Dean B, Pereira E. Surgeons and training time. BMJ Careers. 2011. Available from: http://careers.bmj.com/careers/advice/view-article.html?id=20005162.
63. Herron DM. Establishing and organizing a bariatric surgery programme. In: Inabnet WB, Demaria EJ, Ikramuddin S, editors. Laparoscopic bariatric surgery. Philadelphia: Lippincott Williams & Wilkins; 2005. p. 23–31.
64. Birkmeyer NJ, Dimick JB, Share D, Hawasli A, English WJ, Genaw J, et al. Hospital complication rates with bariatric surgery in Michigan. JAMA. 2010;304:435–42.
65. DeSmidt B. Medicare drops centre of excellence program in bariatric surgery. The Pipeline. 2013. Available from: http://www.advisory.com/research/technology-insights/the-pipeline/2013/10/medicare-drops-center-of-excellence-program-in-bariatric-surgery.
66. Micheal Griffin S, Raimes SA, Jon S. Oesophagogastric surgery. Edinburgh/New York: Elsevier; 2014. p. 358–80. 978-0-7020-4962-0.

Chapter 8
Teaching Advanced Laparoscopic Skills in Urological Surgery

Clare Sweeney and Alan McNeill

Background

Urology has always been a pioneering specialty in minimally access surgery, with the first attempt at cystoscopy made in 1807 by Philipp Bozzini, however it was impractical and it was not until 1878 that the first working cystoscope was presented by Nitze/Leiter. The Hopkins rod lens system was patented in 1959 and revolutionized urological surgery. Hopkins in combination with Karl Storz created modern cystoscopes and simultaneous developments in fibre-optic technology facilitated the development of flexible instruments [1]. However it was not until 1990 that the first laparoscopic nephrectomy was performed, 5 years after the first laparoscopic cholecystectomy was carried out and 15 years after the first laparoscopic salpingectomy [2].

Since then the role of minimally access surgery in urology has increased exponentially. The indications for a laparoscopic approach are continually expanding with skills acquisition and improvements in technology. Laparoscopic radical nephrectomy is now the gold standard treatment of clinically T2 renal tumours [3] and both hospital stay and blood loss have been reduced through the introduction of laparoscopic radical prostatectomy [4]. The most commonly performed laparoscopic urological surgeries are nephrectomy, prostatectomy, and pyeloplasty. However there is interest in expansion of the role of minimal access surgery to include even more complex surgery with higher associated morbidity such as partial nephrectomy and cystectomy. The challenge remains to perform an equivalent

C. Sweeney, BMedSci, MBChB, MEd, FRCS(Urol)
Department of Urology, NHS Taysidem Ninewells Hospital, Dundee, Scotland, UK
e-mail: clare.sweeney@nhslothian.scot.nhs.uk

A. McNeill, BMedSci,BMBS,FRCSEd/Eng,FRCS (✉)
Department of Urology, Western General Hospital, Crewe Road, Edinburgh EH4 2XU, UK
e-mail: alan.mcneill@luht.scot.nhs.uk

N. Francis et al. (eds.), *Training in Minimal Access Surgery*,
DOI 10.1007/978-1-4471-6494-4_8

technical and oncological operation laparoscopically, whilst minimising post operative pain and its associated complications thus reducing hospital stay.

Such complex surgery requires extensive technical skills training. Learning the professional practice of surgery traditionally took place entirely within the 'swampy lowlands of practice' [5]. Surgical trainees undertook an apprenticeship working long hours over several years, developing their skills on real patients, at the feet of their masters. Formal postgraduate education was limited and there was no defined surgical curriculum or end point. Training in this fashion has been described as 'magpie like', accruing tips and techniques from each trainer. The quantity of procedures a trainee had performed unsupervised was often the most important measure of surgical skills development in the UK. Such arrangements resulted in trainees with a wealth of independent operating experience, perhaps without regard for the patient outcome.

The expansion of major urological minimal access surgery has coincided with extensive changes in the structure of surgical training. In 1993, *Hospital doctors: Training for the future: the report of the working group on specialist medical training* was published [6]. It became known as the Calman report and would radically reform higher specialist training. Before the Calman reforms of higher surgical training, trainees spent an average of 30,000 h in training posts before becoming consultants. In 1996 the implementation of the Calman reforms to surgical training in the UK reduced this to 18,000–21,000 h [7] and more recently the changes following Modernising Medical Careers and European Working Time Directive (EWTD) have reduced this further to an expected 6–8000 h [8]. If we are to train competent surgeons in one fifth of the time it used to take it is clear we can no longer rely on experiential learning alone to develop expertise.

Such marked reductions in the duration of training and volume of independent operating, begs the question how will surgical trainees develop their skills and make the transition from novice to expert? We know from Simon and Chase that future experts gradually acquire patterns and knowledge about how to react in situations as a direct consequence of their continued experience in the domain [9]. The number of procedures performed a year by a surgeon has been shown to be an independent predictor of outcome [10]. However trainees no longer have seemingly endless training opportunities and expertise will have to be acquired from a shorter, more intense training programme.

However, reduction in working hours is not the only challenge that face current trainees trying to develop expertise in minimal access surgery. In 2000 the NHS Plan outlined the need for a service led by trained doctors, not by trainees [11]. Profound changes in healthcare culture with a move towards patients as consumers of healthcare have necessitated major changes in training. It is no longer appropriate to practice on patients and subject them to the Proficiency-gain curve of the trainee.

It is clear therefore that a multi-modal approach is required to gain expertise in complex psychomotor skills required for increasingly complex laparoscopic procedures. In learning laparoscopy trainees must convert a two dimensional video image into three dimensions in their mind, adjust to loss of haptic feedback from tissue and adapt to counter-intuitive hand movements in a small space. The Joint Committee on Surgical Training (JCST) anticipate that most urology trainees should be able to perform a laparoscopic nephrectomy with minimal assistance by the end of their training, but they accept that currently this is aspirational [12]. Only a small proportion of urological surgeons will go on to provide more complex laparoscopic procedures such as pyeloplasty and prostatectomy. With increasing experience in minimal access surgery, more difficult cases are being performed laparoscopically, e.g. laparoscopic radical nephrectomy for T2/3 renal tumours, whereas most T1 renal tumours are undergoing partial nephrectomy – the so-called easy laparoscopic cases are disappearing for trainees [13].

Theory and Practice/Educational Principles: How Do We Learn New Skills?

The skills necessary for minimal access surgery are fundamentally different from traditional open surgery and the speed of acquisition does not differ between residents and experienced surgeons [14]. Laparoscopy provides an ideal model to investigate how people progress from novice to expert. The first stage of gaining expertise is cognitive, learning the steps of the procedure, the next is associative, learning to perform these steps and the third is autonomous, when the actions are automatic and the clinician no longer has to think about how to carry out the procedure.

Expert Performance

Ericsson recognised that whilst experience is necessary it is alone not enough to ensure expert performance. "Nobody becomes an outstanding professional without experience, but extensive experience does not invariably lead people to become experts" [9]. That is, straightforward repetition of a task is ineffective unless it is underpinned by a drive to learn and improve [15]. He went on to argue that whilst most professionals reach an acceptable level of proficiency within a relatively short time frame and maintain this level of mediocrity for the rest of their careers, some individuals continue to improve and are eventually recognised as experts. Performance increases gradually and most elite performers need a minimum of 10 years intense involvement in a domain to attain high levels of performance.

Acquisition of expertise requires sustained deliberate practice. Deliberate practice is achieved when trainees are instructed to improve some aspect of their performance in a procedure, are offered immediate detailed feedback and have ample opportunities to improve their performance gradually by performing the same or similar procedures repeatedly. Without this, an acceptable level of performance is attained after a limited period of training and skills tend to become automated. Therefore the challenge for surgeons is to "avoid the arrested development associated with automaticity" [15]. Performance continues to improve as long as training sessions are limited to around an hour. The best groups of expert musicians spend around 4 h a day in solitary practice. Masters in any domain better anticipate future situations and it has been shown that chess masters can play blindfolded [9]. This perhaps can be extrapolated to masters in a surgical technique for example an expert laparoscopic surgeon will know where the tip of a needle is even if they cannot see it.

Automaticity

Whilst the aim of training in laparoscopic urological surgery is to provide a safe and effective level of performance certain aspects of a procedure should be rendered automatic. Surgeons should be able to throw a knot without thinking about it, whether they are operating open or laparoscopically if the procedure requires it. During the first phase of learning novices concentrate on avoiding mistakes, with more experience gross mistakes are rarer and learners no longer need to concentrate as hard. After a limited period of training an acceptable standard is met at which point some actions become automated. Trainees execute these skills smoothly and without apparent effort. Ericsson points out that as a consequence of automation performers lose conscious control over execution of those skills making internal modifications difficult [9], performance reaches a stable plateau. For most surgeons tying a knot is automatic and trying to break it down into component parts to teach it can be challenging. Laparoscopic suturing should be the easy bit of an operation as it can be practiced until it is automatic in the box trainer before suturing in the stressful environment of a live operation.

Zone of Proximal Development

Surgical trainees operate within Vygotsky's 'zone of proximal development', that is the distance between the actual developmental level of the trainee and the level of potential development as determined through problem solving in collaboration with more capable peers; it is the space where guided learning takes place [16]. The zone can be populated with all the tools trainees need to develop expertise such as expert tuition and simulation. Vygotsky recognised that instruction is only good when it proceeds ahead of development, that is a good trainer provides help when needed but fades into the background when the trainee becomes independent [17]. During the final stages of learning a technique assistance can be counterproductive, as it interferes with the process of internalization.

It is clear that skills acquisition requires an orderly and deliberate approach, a curriculum for learning. Lack of an effective curriculum prevents learning gains from being consolidated and developed, and the absence of regular reinforcement results in the loss of many recently acquired skills. Performance must be sustained and distributed not massed, which builds in an element of overlearning [15]. There is rapid decay of knowledge following massed practice.

Laparoscopy in Urology

Current Status of Minimal Access Surgery in Urology

In 2013 in England & Wales, 7591 nephrectomies were reported to the British Association of Urological Surgeons nephrectomy audit by 341 consultants from 145 centres [18]. It has been estimated that 40 % of all urologists perform nephrectomies. The median number of nephrectomies performed per consultant was 16 and the median per centre was 39. Of these nephrectomies 71.3 % or 5413, were documented as laparoscopic procedures making laparoscopic nephrectomy the most commonly performed laparoscopic urological procedure. Most are carried out for malignancy, T1b – T3 renal tumours and nephro-ureterectomy for upper tract transitional cell carcinoma (TCC), but 15 % are carried out for benign disease, so called 'simple nephrectomy'. It is recommended that surgeons and trainees wishing to commence laparoscopic training should start with upper tract surgery. From a training perspective the simplest laparoscopic nephrectomies are not for benign disease but for T1 tumours. Whilst the current generation of laparoscopic surgeons gained much of their experience through removing kidneys for small tumours most of these are now treated by partial nephrectomy and so the relatively 'easy' cases are less frequent.

Fewer laparoscopic pyeloplasties are performed each year and as such only a few surgeons should be performing these procedures, typically 1/2 per centre. Pyeloplasty often falls to the laparoscopic renal surgeon and whilst surgeons require all the skills necessary to perform laparoscopic nephrectomy they also need another level of technical mastery for pyeloplasty, that of laparoscopic suturing. As renal surgeons they may not be performing other operations that require laparoscopic suturing and if they are performing less than 1 pyeloplasty a month they must be motivated to continue regular deliberate practice in a box trainer in between cases to maintain this skill.

In the same British Association of Urological Surgeons (BAUS) audit in 2013, 3695 radical prostatectomies were carried out in 62 centres by 130 consultants in England [19]. 30 % of these (1113) were laparoscopic, 49 % (1825) were robotic and 13 % were open (490), whilst the approach was not recorded in 245 cases. The median number performed per consultant was 16 and the median per centre was 38. Whilst it is recommended that all trainees have some experience in laparoscopic upper tract surgery only a few experts will offer more complex laparoscopic procedures such as prostatectomy. High volume centres seem to have better outcomes. Laparoscopic radical prostatectomy is a uniquely challenging procedure for which training in the UK is limited to a few centres. The procedure demands an extremely high level of laparoscopic surgical competency. Proper training and mentorship can facilitate learning laparoscopic radical prostatectomy and reproducible the results.

Setting up a service to provide even more complex laparoscopic urological surgeries remains in its infancy in most UK centres. In contrast to other major urological oncology operations audited in 2013, 60 % of 1024 radical cystectomies reported were carried out open and 15 % were carried out robotically (i.e including diversion) in England [20]. 52 % of partial nephrectomies were carried out laparoscopically in this time period. Surgeons must have the appropriate expertise for this technically demanding procedure with inherent risk of positive surgical margin, haemorrhage and renal dysfunction associated with warm ischaemia. Published evidence comes from highly specialised units where clinicians have undertaken a large number of laparoscopic partial nephrectomies [21].

Mentorship

Trainee laparoscopic surgeons learn in a new style apprenticeship under the guidance of a mentor. Learning minimal access surgery is now an integral part of the curriculum for urology trainees and one aim of the Joint Committee on Surgical Training (JCST) in the UK is that all trainees will be able to perform laparoscopic nephrectomy by the time they have completed their training [12]. As a consequence of the rapid uptake of laparoscopic techniques, established consultants as well as trainees have been learning complex laparoscopic surgery. Whereas there is an established subspecialty curriculum in place for urology trainees, initially consultants were learning from other relatively inexperienced laparoscopic surgeons in a somewhat *ad hoc* manner. For this reason BAUS published mentorship guidelines to ensure that only consultants carrying out laparoscopic procedures on a regular basis could act as mentors [22]. The guidelines lay out the responsibilities of both mentor and mentee in the training process.

Mentors for laparoscopic nephrectomy should fulfill the following criteria:

- Have performed >50 laparoscopic nephrectomies independently as a consultant
- Submit the results to the annual BAUS laparoscopic nephrectomy audit
- Ensure the trainee has:
  - notified his medical director and lead clinician of this new development
  - is aware of NICE guidelines on laparoscopic nephrectomy
  - has attended a BAUS delines on laparoscopic nephrectomhas an undertaking from colleagues to refer appropriate cases
  - limits his indications to nephrectomy until he is deemed competent in that procedure
  - performed at least one laparoscopic nephrectomy s deemed competent in that procedure

Similarly they recommend that mentors for more complex procedures should fulfil additional criteria:

- For pyeloplasty: to have performed >20 cases independently as a consultant and to have submitted the results to the BAUS section of endourology pelvi-ureteric junction (PUJ) audit
- For partial nephrectomy: to have performed >100 laparoscopic nephrectomies and 20 partial nephrectomies independently as a consultant and to have submitted the results to the BAUS Laparoscopic Nephrectomy audit.
- For radical prostatectomy: to have performed >100 cases independently as a consultant and to have submitted the results to the BAUS section of oncology audit.

Novices who wish to learn urological laparoscopy must complete the following steps:

- Complete a wis'olaboratory and develop facilities to practice at home
- Complete an animal-based cwet; laboratory course
- Watch live procedures in the context of demonstrations i.e., a masterclass
- Attend a high-volume centre to watch designated cases; and the proposed theatre team to visit a high-volume centre to learn all aspects of surgery
- Identify a mentor
- Start practicing laparoscopic nephrectomy with the mentor
- At the end of the training period do several procedures independently, observed by an experienced laparoscopic surgeon
- Audit their results; submit the results to the BAUS annual laparoscopic nephrectomy audit
- Aim to do at least 12 marker cases a year

Modular Training

One approach to training complex minimal access surgery is to break the surgery down into small blocks or modules. This allows novices to gain experience under close supervision from a mentor within a patient-centered environment. Modular training is in line with educational principles of sustained, distributed, deliberate practice. Trainees concentrate on the module appropriate to their level without trying to complete the whole operation. Once each module has been mastered they can put the modules together. We know that the optimum duration for concentration is around an hour; so when concentrating on learning the more difficult modules, such as hilar dissection, trainees might not do the 'easier' modules leading up to it. In keeping with educational principles it is important that mentors step back at the right time as continued presence can hinder consolidation. It has been suggested that laparoscopic nephrectomy be broken down into 23 steps, which can be grouped into 5 modules [23]. These are:

1. Positioning, trocar placement and closure
2. Division of adhesions and mobilisation of colon/duodenum, elevation of ureter and specimen extraction

3. Lower pole mobilisation and identification of renal hilum
4. Dissection of renal hilum and division of artery and vein, upper pole mobilisation and adrenalectomy on left
5. Upper pole mobilisation and adrenalectomy on right

Similarly laparoscopic radical prostatectomy can be divided into 12 steps and 5 modules [24]. These are:

1. Trocar placement, development of pre-peritoneal space, incision of endo-pelvic fascia and division of pubo-prostatic ligaments
2. Pelvic lymphadenectomy and anterior/lateral bladder neck dissection, 3 and 9 o'clock sutures
3. Ligation of dorsal venous complex, posterior bladder neck dissection, division of vas and dissection of seminal vesicles, dissection of posterior surface and prostatic pedicles, bladder neck closure and 11 and 1 o'clock sutures
4. Apical dissection and urethra-vesical anastomosis
5. Nerve-sparing procedure

After a period of camera holding and assisting in laparoscopic prostatectomy it is estimated that trainees must perform around 40 procedures before being considered competent. However this is dependent on the individual and whilst the learning curve is estimated at 40–100 cases surgeons continue to improve, even after 300 cases [25].

Assessing Competence

Currently established consultants who wish to learn laparoscopy will need to be signed off by their mentor in accordance with above guidelines. In order to become accredited at the end of the designated training period they must perform several laparoscopic procedures independently whilst being observed by an experienced laparoscopic surgeon. In addition they commit to performing at least 12 procedures a year and auditing their results, both locally and submitting their results to the national BAUS audit.

Current trainees undergoing laparoscopic training are used to a more rigorous assessment model. As part of the new higher surgical curriculum introduced in the UK in 2007 trainees and trainers alike were introduced to workplace-based assessments. Workplace-based assessments are described as a formative assessment tool to support learning and act as an adjunct to the surgical logbook. They aim to assess the top level of Miller's pyramid that is what the trainee 'does' in the clinical setting [26]. Trainees who are currently nearing completion of training should therefore be able to provide a portfolio of evidence documenting their progression and ultimately competence to perform a laparoscopic nephrectomy. Currently these assessments only evaluate nephrectomy skills suggesting that more complex operations such as laparoscopic radical prostatectomy are considered too challenging for higher surgical training and should be developed after receipt of a Certificate of Completion of Training. However, as more and more of these operations are carried out by minimal access techniques more and more trainees will gain significant experience in certain modules of the procedure, which should be subject to assessment in the same manner.

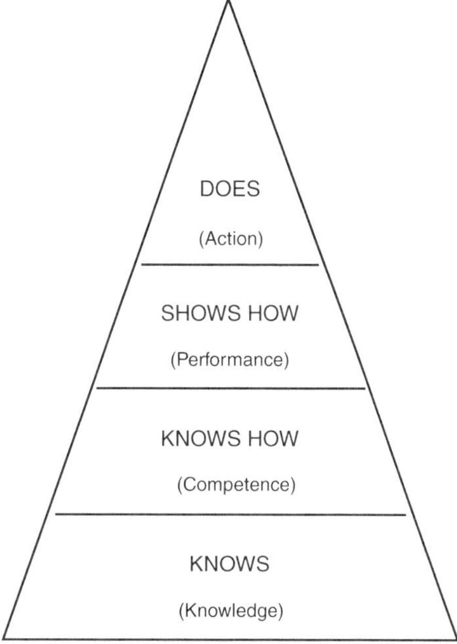

Fig. 8.1 Miller's pyramid, a framework for clinical assessment (With permission from Wolters Kluwer Health, Inc, from: Miller [26])

There is an argument that there should be a higher level of Miller's pyramid – what the trainee 'does well'.

Over the past 5 years we have developed a wealth of experience with procedure-based assessments in the higher surgical training curriculum and this could easily be utilised to incorporate a more formal assessment into the mentorship programme for established consultants learning laparoscopy (Fig. 8.1).

Robotic Surgery

Given the particular technical challenges of complex laparoscopic urological surgery some centres have moved instead to robotic-assisted surgery. Robotic surgery does not demand the same level of laparoscopic skill, it provides a 3D image, removes counter-intuitive hand movements and filters tremor. As a result it is even more precise than laparoscopic surgery and the expectation is that functional outcomes should improve. Unfortunately the costs are prohibitive and it is only economically viable to high volume centres.

Training the Team

Performing complex minimal access surgery requires a new skills set, not just for the main operator, but for the whole surgical team. Theatre staff must familiarize themselves with the equipment used and should know the steps of the procedure to better anticipate the surgeon's needs. One or two trained surgical assistants are also required. A trained surgical practitioner can provide consistency in this role and become a linchpin for the team. As trained assistants they are familiar with the steps of the procedure, all the specialist equipment and liaise with suppliers. We have found it useful when training and indeed setting up a laparoscopic service for the whole team to visit an established centre, usually that of the mentor, prior to starting a new procedure. This gives an opportunity for the team to learn by legitimate peripheral participation and by observing the established team, asking questions and identifying potential pitfalls prior to encountering them in their own unit.

Conclusion

The role of minimal access surgery in the field of urological surgery is ever expanding. Advances in equipment and extensive skills development have led to more and more procedures being carried out laparoscopically. This brings advantages for patients, but also particular challenges in technical skills training. We would recommend that learning the technical skills required for laparoscopic urological surgery take place within a defined curriculum. Training requires observation, sustained deliberate practice, including a combination of high and low fidelity simulation, and a modular approach to real life surgery that is appropriately mentored. For established consultants and post CCT trainees we would recommend a whole team approach to learning with a mentorship programme to ensure patient safety and quality control. Once surgeons have been signed off they must maintain their skills by performing a minimum number of cases per annum and participating in ongoing appraisal by auditing their own results and submitting to the national audit.

References

1. Shah J. Endoscopy through the ages. BJUI. 2002;89:645–52.
2. Clayman RV, Kavoussi LR, Soper NJ, et al. Laparoscopic nephrectomy: initial case report. J Urol. 1991;146:278–82.
3. Ljungberg B, Bensalah K, Bex A, et al. Guidelines on renal cell carcinoma. European Association of Urology. Eur Urol. 2013;67(5):913–24.
4. Finkelstein J, Eckersberger E, Sadri H, et al. Open versus laparoscopic versus robot-assisted laparoscopic prostatectomy: the European and US experience. Rev Urol. 2010;12(1):35–43.
5. Schon D. Preparing professionals for the demands of practice p3 in educating the reflective practitioner. San Francisco: Jossey-Bass Inc Publishers; 1987.
6. Department of Health. Hospital Doctors: training for the future. The Report of the Working Group on Specialist Medical Training. London: Department of Health; 1993.
7. Cresswell B, Marron C, Hawkins W, et al. Optimising working hours to provide quality in training and patient safety a position statement by The Association of Surgeons in Training. 2009.
8. Chikwe J, deSouza AC, Pepper JR. No time to train the surgeons. BMJ. 2004;328(7437):418–9.
9. Ericsson KA. Deliberate practice and the acquisition and maintenance of expert performance in medicine and related domains. Acad Med. 2004;79(10):S70–81.

10. Davenport K, Timoney AG, Keeley Jr FX, Joyce AD, Downey P. A 3-year review of the British Association of Urological Surgeons Section of Endourology Laparoscopic Nephrectomy Audit. BJUI. 2006;97:333–7.
11. Department of Health. 'The NHS Plan' Department of Health, London; 2000.
12. Joint Committee on Surgical Training. Guidelines for the award of a CCT in Urology. 2012. http://www.jcst.org/quality-assurance/documents/cct-guidelines/urology-cct-guidelines.
13. Imamura M, McLennan S, Lapitan MC, et al. The UCAN Systematic Review Reference Group and the EAU Guideline Group for renal cell carcinoma. Systematic review of clinical effectiveness of surgical management for localized renal cell carcinoma. 2011. University of Aberdeen, Academic Urology Unit: www.uroweb.org/.
14. Stolzenberg J, Rabenalt R, do M, Horn LC, Liatsikos EN. Modular training for residents with no prior experience with open pelvic surgery in endoscopic extraperitoneal radical prostatectomy. Eur Urol. 2005;49:491–500.
15. Kneebone R. Evaluating clinical simulations for learning procedural skills: a theory-based approach. Acad Med. 2005;80(6):549–53.
16. Vygotsky LS. Thought and language. Cambridge, MA: Harvard University Press; 1962.
17. Wood D. How children think and learn. 2nd ed. Oxford: Blackwell; 1998.
18. BAUS Section of Oncology, Analyses of Nephrectomy Dataset Jan 1st – 31st Dec 2013. June 2014.
19. BAUS Section of Oncology, Analyses of Prostatectomy Dataset Jan 1st – 31st Dec 2012. June 2013.
20. BAUS Section of Oncology, Analyses of Cystectomy Dataset Jan 1st – Dec 31st. June 2014.
21. Gill IS, Martin SF, Desai MM, et al. Comparative analysis of laparoscopic versus open partial nephrectomy for renal tumours in 200 patients. J Urol. 2003;170(1):64–8.
22. Keeley FX, Rimington P, Timoney AG, McClinton S. BAUS laparoscopic mentorship guidelines. BAUS. 2007;100(2):247–8.
23. Stewart GD, Phipps S, Little B, et al. Description and validation of a modular training system for laparoscopic nephrectomy. J Endourol. 2012;26(11):1512–7.
24. Stolzenburg J, Schwaibold H, Bhanot SM, et al. Modular surgical training for endoscopic extraperitoneal radical prostatectomy. BJUI. 2005;96:1022–7.
25. Martina GR, Giumelli P, Scuzzarella S, et al. Laparoscopic extraperitoneal radical prostatectomy – learning curve of a laparoscopy naive urologist in a community hospital. Urology. 2005;65:959–63.
26. Miller G. The assessment of clinical skills/competence/performance. Acad Med. 1990;65(9): S63–7.

Chapter 9
Training for New Techniques and Robotic Surgery in Minimal Access Surgery

Jung-Myun Kwak and Sungsoo Park

Introduction

Laparoscopic surgery, which was regarded as an innovative technique over the past two decades, is now more often considered "traditional" or "conventional" in many comparison studies. The growing enthusiasm for even less invasive surgical techniques has led laparoscopic surgeons to try to reduce the number of skin incisions or even avoid them altogether, with single incision laparoscopic surgery (SILS) and natural orifice transluminal endoscopic surgery (NOTES) emerging as experimental alternatives to conventional laparoscopic techniques [1–3]. These methods are becoming increasingly popular among surgeons and the field is expanding. Development of new techniques and technological advances in laparoscopes, instruments, and ports have enhanced the potential for use of SILS and NOTES in a wide variety of surgical procedures, and since Kaouk et al. reported the first successful series of robot-assisted SILS in humans in 2009, there has been a growing interest in development and application of robot-assisted SILS in several surgical specialties [4].

Robotic surgery is increasingly implemented to overcome the technical drawbacks and steep performance- or proficiency-gain curve of traditional laparoscopic surgery. Among the perceived advantages of robotic surgery are the

J.-M. Kwak, MD, PhD
Division of Colorectal Surgery, Department of Surgery, Korea University Anam Hospital, Korea University College of Medicine/MIS & Robotic Surgery Center, Korea University Medical Center, Inchon-ro 73, Seongbuk-gu, Seoul 136-705, South Korea
e-mail: jmkwak@korea.ac.kr

S. Park, MD, PhD (✉)
Division of Upper GI Surgery, Department of Surgery, Korea University Anam Hospital, Korea University College of Medicine/ MIS & Robotic Surgery Center, Korea University Medical Center, Inchon-ro 73, Seongbuk-gu, Seoul 136-705, South Korea
e-mail: kugspss@korea.ac.kr

N. Francis et al. (eds.), *Training in Minimal Access Surgery*,
DOI 10.1007/978-1-4471-6494-4_9

three-dimensional vision, the availability of seven degrees of freedom of movement that truly mimics the movements of the surgeon's hands, a lack of tremor, and the ergonomics of the robotic surgical system. The number and variety of robotic surgical procedures continues to grow, and clinical outcomes are now sufficiently mature to demonstrate safety, efficiency, and reproducibility of some procedures, as well as addressing oncologic and functional outcomes [5–7].

However, at present, there are no standard guidelines for training or safe adoption of robotic techniques. To keep pace with the recent technical and technological advances in minimal access surgery (MAS), training and credentialing paradigms are shifting from traditional mentor-trainee tutorships towards standardized objective and, ideally, safer training programmes. There is a growing consensus that education in MAS should be expanded and begin outside the operating theatre, and that more objective assessment of a surgeon's skills should be introduced to ensure quality of care [8]. Separately, supplementary education for surgeons who have already completed training is also necessary. Designing a training programme to allow experienced surgeons to safely and efficiently implement new technologies and state-of-the-art surgical techniques is essential.

This chapter describes education and training modalities for new MAS and robotic surgery techniques that will support establishment of optimal training programs.

Simulation-Based Training

The adoption of any new technique or new technology comes with the potential risk of injury to the patient. The evolving field of MAS and the need for patient safety requires surgical training by standardized curricula with simulation-based components. Preclinical simulation-based training has been proposed as a useful means of training, and should be considered before new surgical techniques or technologies are applied to actual patient care [9]. The American Board of Surgery now requires that all general surgery graduates provide documentation of successful completion of Fundamentals of Laparoscopic Surgery (FLS) course before sitting for board certification exams [10]. The FLS course is a comprehensive web-based education module that includes a hands-on skills training component and an assessment tool designed to supply fundamental knowledge and teach the physiology and technical skills required for basic laparoscopic surgery. The program features a simulation-based skills laboratory with uniform metrics and assessment criteria.

In addition, the literature suggests that for complex surgical procedures, simulation outside the operating theatre in specially equipped training facilities, such as animal or surgical skills laboratories, may improve the performance- or proficiency-gain curve [11–13]. Traditional and innovative simulation-based training methods that encompass both surgical tasks and skills without risk to patients should be considered when establishing a training programme.

Knowledge Development

Before implementing a new technique or technology, it is essential for the surgeon to gain basic knowledge of appropriate patient selection and indications, proper pre-operative preparation, patient positioning and trocar placement, types of complications and their management, as well as to understand the new devices and equipment. Trainees should be fully aware of procedural steps for a new technique.

In this regard, the manufacturer of the da Vinci robotic surgical system has established training centers worldwide to provide an introduction to the robotic surgical system and preparation for its use, as basic product training before clinical training. Thus, trainees have the opportunity to acquire knowledge and understanding of the technology, devices, basic functions and limitations of the system.

Structured Inanimate Skills Tasks

Inanimate models (box trainers) are available for minimal access surgery, and can be helpful to trainees. An inherent problem with training on these models, however, is that the training is heavily dependent on the trainee. Unless a mentor is available to monitor a given trainee's progress on an inanimate trainer, which is usually not the case, the trainees are left to assess their own surgical skills, and overestimation of skill acquisition is likely.

Virtual Reality Simulator

A virtual reality (VR) simulator is a useful training tool, particularly for minimal access surgical techniques and robotic surgery. It has now been proven with level 1 evidence that VR simulation-based training can improve operating room performance among surgical residents who are preparing for laparoscopic cholecystectomy [14]. In contrast to the inanimate trainer, a VR simulator provides a computer-based platform with artificially generated virtual environments. It can also provide a virtual instructor and apply standardized metrics to assess performance and identify errors and areas of improvement to promote proficiency.

A number of factors in the current surgical environment have prompted the development of simulators. Concerns about operative times and economic issues can limit a surgical trainee's experience in the operating room, and having the novice surgeon achieve a certain level of competency before participating in actual operating room procedures has been proposed as method of improving efficiency and safety in the operating room [15–17]. Other issues surrounding surgical training include medico-legal concerns, limits to the number of work hours permitted for trainees, and ethical considerations related to a trainee learning basic skills on humans and animals [18]. Since developments in computer technology have now led to the introduction of VR simulators that allow standardized and objective training and evaluation of surgical skills, many of these issues can potentially be avoided [19].

Robotic surgical training presents some unique challenges in comparison to laparoscopic training. While good hand-eye-coordination is necessary for laparoscopic surgery, robotic techniques require different skills involving foot-hand-eye coordination in order for the surgeon to manage the robotic console. Dry laboratory practice with robotic instruments for exercise of these psychomotor skills requires the purchase of a separate robot system for training purposes. Robotic surgical training with a live animal model or a fresh frozen cadaver is generally too expensive for regular training practice. Furthermore, traditional supervised interventions on patients are potentially hazardous during robotic surgical training. During conventional laparoscopic surgery, the mentoring surgeon is adjacent to the trainee, has the same view of the procedure, and can take over at any given moment where patient safety may be compromised. However, as only one surgeon can be at an operating console (although some alternatives are discussed below), this is usually not the case in robotic procedures [20].

Therefore, the use of a VR simulator is an appealing option for robotic surgical training. The VR simulator provides surgeons with safe and extensive training in preparation for surgery on patients, and presently it offers the greatest potential for improved surgical skills. Surgical skills training in a virtual environment has a significant learning effect and the learned skills are consistent with and transferable to actual robotic procedures [21–23].

There are several commercially available high-fidelity VR simulators. The Ross™, manufactured by Simulated Surgical Systems (Williamsville, NY, USA), has both validated basic orientation modules and basic skill modules. It is the only robotic surgery simulator featuring full-length surgical procedures and has a patent-pending procedural task for robotic prostatectomy. Other procedural components are also being developed [24].

The dV-Trainer™ by Mimic Technologies (Seattle, WA, USA) was the first commercially available simulator for robotic surgery. Several validation studies have demonstrated face, content, construct, and concurrent validity (chapter 2) of this VR simulator [25–28]. Through a partnership with Intuitive Surgical, Inc. (Sunnyvale, CA, USA), the manufacturer of the da Vinci robotic surgical system, the dV-Trainer™ uses the da Vinci robot kinematics, instrument design, and vision display. The dV-Trainer™ software is suitable for use within the robotic console, allowing virtual tasks to be performed in a real-life environment. There are more than 50 exercise modules, but currently there are no procedural components.

The da Vinci Skills Simulator™ was presented by Intuitive Surgical in partnership with Mimic Technologies to integrate the software of the dV-Trainer™ into the da Vinci Si console through the backpack. Thus, there is no actual hardware for this VR simulator, and the actual da Vinci Si console becomes the hardware. As with dV-Trainer™, there are no procedural components.

Surgical Tasks in a Live Animal Model

The live animal simulation model has been considered one of the most important components of training in robotic surgery and has been incorporated in several courses [29–31]. Although the anatomy is different, operating on an animal model provides good replication of the visco-elastic properties of human tissue and its response to manipulation, dissection, ligation, and other operative manoeuvres. However, live animal simulation models are costly and veterinary assistance and separate equipment and location are required. Furthermore, it may raise ethical concerns.

Nonetheless, the live animal model is still considered the simulation model with the highest fidelity in terms of close replication of intra-operative conditions, even as wet laboratories are limited and many surgical trainees will complete their training without an opportunity to operate on an animal model.

Surgical Tasks in the Fresh Frozen Cadaver

The fresh frozen cadaver simulation model has the advantage of presenting real human anatomy and can be useful for procedural training. Surgical anatomy, tissue consistency, and anatomical planes are usually well preserved, and participants report high levels of satisfaction [32].

However, such a training programme is not easily reproducible, and is costly, requiring special preparation and separate equipment, as with the live animal simulation model. Another limitation is the lack of in vivo physiology such as bleeding and actual tissue compliance. There is a paucity of studies exploring the true effectiveness of fresh frozen cadaver training [33].

Proctoring

Proctoring is a process involving observation by another, preferably more experienced, surgeon during the initial phase of the performance-gain curve of a trainee in order to assess the trainee's knowledge and skills in the use of a new equipment or technique. A review regarding proctoring underlined its importance for robotic surgery and institutional credentialing and addressed its medico-legal aspects. Although extended proctorship is an expensive way of training, it provides a relatively safe way of introducing a new technique and it prevents surgeons from beginning to perform new procedures before they have mastered the techniques [34].

Mentoring

Mentoring, on the other hand, is a form of training whereby the experienced surgeon scrubs in or supervises a procedure with the intention of guiding the trainee and assisting with the acquisition of new skills during the steep part of the proficiency-gain curve. Therefore, it should ideally be independent of assessment, performance review, or evaluation. Mentoring helps trainee perceive strengths and blind spots, overcome difficulties, enable self-challenge, discuss problems and fulfill goals [35].

Mentoring during the actual performance of a robotic operation can be carried out in several ways. The mentor can closely observe the trainee while the trainee is performing an operation, give verbal instruction, and take control of the operation when necessary. Another option is the use of a mentoring console, when one is available. The mentoring console is a second console that allows the surgeon and the trainee to collaborate via either of two collaborative modes, a swap mode, which allows the mentor and the trainee to operate simultaneously and actively swap control of the robot arms; and a nudge mode, which allows both operators to have control over two robot arms. The nudge mode seems to be particularly useful for guiding the trainee's hands during certain steps of an operation [36].

Video Clinics

Video technology is now commonly used as a source of teaching and training in various aspects of medical education. The advantages of incorporating video into web-based education include ease of access, cost-effectiveness, time efficiency, and independent learning. Many surgical societies now offer some web-based teaching materials on their home pages. Illustrative surgery is selected in advance and the education can be also planned ahead of time [37–39].

Watching an unedited video with the expert surgeon as a part of a mentoring process and discussing the procedure point-by-point is one of the most effective training methods, particularly for a surgeon in the proficiency-gain curve. The trainees can choose illustrative cases of their own and focus a discussion on educational moments, regardless of the actual time that the surgery took place. This kind of video teaching/learning programme still requires scheduling coordination, and it can be very time-consuming. It can be useful to offer this mode of training as part of a short intensive training course. Sending a video to a mentor or watching a video together online is alternative option to save time and travel.

Live Surgery Demonstrations

Rapid advances in technology, the drive to improve quality and safety, and the dissemination of information about new tools, equipment, and state-of-the-art surgical techniques have led to the development of courses that include live surgery demonstrations from around the world.

There are several ways to implement live surgery demonstrations. Real-time presence in the operating room to observe an operation performed by an expert surgeon is an important component for a robotic surgery training programme or for learning other new surgical techniques [40]. In this scenario, it is possible to communicate freely with the expert surgeon and observe other important factors such as patient positioning, trocar placement, communication and teamwork, and decision-making.

Live surgery demonstrations may also be broadcast to professional meetings and this option has grown in popularity, although there has been some criticism regarding ethical issues and possible compromise of patient safety caused by the added stress on the surgeon and surgical team. Nonetheless, live surgery demonstration by this method can be an effective educational tool and it can confirm the quality of the surgical procedure [41, 42]. Observing live surgery provides an experience that allows critical peer-to-peer discussion to make significant points of the procedure more clear.

Conclusions

Designing competence-based training curricula for the new techniques in MAS and robotic surgery remains a challenge. However, with the considerable increase in the number of centres that are adopting robotic surgery and other new techniques, the need for uniform, certified curricula has also rapidly increased. At present, there remains a lack of validated training tools, and further research in this field needs to be performed in the near future. As the quality of virtual reality simulators for robotic surgery continues to increase, it is expected that this training modality will continue to have an expanding role. It is essential that procedural training is carried out in a step-by-step manner using proctoring, mentoring, video review, and live surgery demonstrations. These options could be combined in a complementary fashion and conducted either face-to-face or by using modern electronic media to save time, travel and to enable increased flexibility. In this way, introduction of new techniques and technologies can be accomplished safely and efficiently, and without compromising patient safety and outcomes.

References

1. Mohan HM, O'Riordan JM, Winter DC. Natural-orifice translumenal endoscopic surgery (NOTES): minimally invasive evolution or revolution? Surg Laparosc Endosc Percutan Tech. 2013;23:244–50.
2. Chukwumah C, Zorron R, Marks JM, Ponsky JL. Current status of natural orifice translumenal endoscopic surgery (NOTES). Curr Probl Surg. 2010;47:630–68.
3. Ahmed I, Ciancio F, Ferrara V, Jorgensen LN, Mann O, Morales-Conde S, Paraskeva P, Vestweber B, Weiss H. Current status of single-incision laparoscopic surgery: European experts' views. Surg Laparosc Endosc Percutan Tech. 2012;22:194–9.
4. Kaouk JH, Goel RK, Haber GP, Crouzet S, Stein RJ. Robotic single-port transumbilical surgery in humans: initial report. BJU Int. 2009;103:366–9.
5. Kwak JM, Kim SH, Kim J, Son DN, Baek SJ, Cho JS. Robotic vs laparoscopic resection of rectal cancer: short-term outcomes of a case-control study. Dis Colon Rectum. 2011;54:151–6.
6. Kim JY, Kim NK, Lee KY, Hur H, Min BS, Kim JH. A comparative study of voiding and sexual function after total mesorectal excision with autonomic nerve preservation for rectal cancer: laparoscopic versus robotic surgery. Ann Surg Oncol. 2012;19:2485–93.
7. Baek SJ, Lee DW, Park SS, Kim SH. Current status of robot-assisted gastric surgery. World J Gastrointest Oncol. 2011;3:137–43.
8. Oropesa I, Sánchez-González P, Lamata P, Chmarra MK, Pagador JB, Sánchez-Margallo JA, Sánchez-Margallo FM, Gómez EJ. Methods and tools for objective assessment of psychomotor skills in laparoscopic surgery. J Surg Res. 2011;171:e81–95.
9. Fried MP, Satava R, Weghorst S, Gallagher AG, Sasaki C, Ross D, Sinanan M, Uribe JI, Zeltsan M, Arora H, Cuellar H. Identifying and reducing errors with surgical simulation. Qual Saf Health Care. 2004;13 Suppl 1:i19–26.
10. The American Board of Surgery Fundamentals of Laparoscopic Surgery course is available at http://www.absurgery.org. Last accessed 20 Aug 2013.
11. Stelzer MK, Abdel MP, Sloan MP, Gould JC. Dry lab practice leads to improved laparoscopic performance in the operating room. J Surg Res. 2009;154:163–6.
12. Scott DJ, Dunnington GL. The new ACS/APDS skills curriculum: moving the learning curve out of the operating room. J Gastrointest Surg. 2008;12:213–21.
13. Scott DJ, Bergen PC, Rege RV, Laycock R, Tesfay ST, Valentine RJ, Euhus DM, Jeyarajah DR, Thompson WM, Jones DB. Laparoscopic training on bench models: better and more cost effective than operating room experience? J Am Coll Surg. 2000;191:272–83.
14. Seymour NE, Gallagher AG, Roman SA, O'Brien MK, Bansal VK, Andersen DK, Satava RM. Virtual reality training improves operating room performance: results of a randomized, double-blinded study. Ann Surg. 2002;236:458–63.
15. Lee BR, Caddedu JA, Janetschek G, Schulam P, Docimo SG, Moore RG, Partin AW, Kavoussi LR. International surgical telemonitoring: our initial experience. Stud Health Technol Inform. 1998;50:41–7.
16. Caddedu JA, Kondraske GV. Human performance testing and simulators. J Endourol. 2007;21:300–4.
17. Rehring ST, Powers K, Jones DB. Integrating simulation in surgery as a teaching tool and credentialing standard. J Gastrointest Surg. 2008;12:222–33.
18. Subramonian K, Muir G. The 'learning curve' in surgery: what is it, how do we measure it and can we influence it? BJU Int. 2004;93:1173–4.
19. Grantcharov TP, Kristiansen VB, Bendix J, Bardram L, Funch-Jensen P. Randomized clinical trial of virtual reality simulation for laparoscopic skills training. Br J Surg. 2004;91:146–50.
20. Abboudi H, Khan MS, Aboumarzouk O, Guru KA, Challacombe B, Dasgupta P, Ahmed K. Current status of validation for robotic surgery simulators – a systematic review. BJU Int. 2013;111:194–205.

21. Brown-Clerk B, Siu KC, Katsavelis D, Lee I, Oleynikov D, Stergiou N. Validating advanced robot-assisted laparoscopic training task in virtual reality. Stud Health Technol Inform. 2008;132:45–9.
22. Mukherjee M, Siu KC, Suh IH, Klutman A, Oleynikov D, Stergiou N. A virtual reality training program for improvement of robotic surgical skills. Stud Health Technol Inform. 2009;142:210–4.
23. Suh IH, Siu KC, Mukherjee M, Monk E, Oleynikov D, Stergiou N. Consistency of performance of robot-assisted surgical tasks in virtual reality. Stud Health Technol Inform. 2009;142:369–73.
24. Lallas CD, Davis JW, Members Of The Society Of Urologic Robotic Surgeons. Robotic surgery training with commercially available simulation systems in 2011: a current review and practice pattern survey from the society of urologic robotic surgeons. J Endourol. 2012;26:283–93.
25. Kenney PA, Wszolek MF, Gould JJ, Libertino JA, Moinzadeh A. Face, content, and construct validity of dV-trainer, a novel virtual reality simulator for robotic surgery. Urology. 2009;73:1288–92.
26. Lendvay TS, Casale P, Sweet R, Peters C. Initial validation of a virtual-reality robotic simulator. J Robot Surg. 2008;2:145–9.
27. Lendvay TS, Casale P, Sweet R, Peters C. VR robotic surgery: randomized blinded study of the dV-Trainer robotic simulator. Stud Health Technol Inform. 2008;132:242–4.
28. Sethi AS, Peine WJ, Mohammadi Y, Sundaram CP. Validation of a novel virtual reality robotic simulator. J Endourol. 2009;23:503–8.
29. Mehrabi A, Yetimoglu CL, Nickkholgh A, Kashfi A, Kienle P, Konstantinides L, Ahmadi MR, Fonouni H, Schemmer P, Friess H, Gebhard MM, Büchler MW, Schmidt J, Gutt CN. Development and evaluation of a training module for the clinical introduction of the da Vinci robotic system in visceral and vascular surgery. Surg Endosc. 2006;20:1376–82.
30. Hanly EJ, Marohn MR, Bachman SL, Talamini MA, Hacker SO, Howard RS, Schenkman NS. Multiservice laparoscopic surgical training using the daVinci surgical system. Am J Surg. 2004;187:309–15.
31. Vlaovic PD, Sargent ER, Boker JR, Corica FA, Chou DS, Abdelshehid CS, White SM, Sala LG, Chu F, Le T, Clayman RV, McDougall EM. Immediate impact of an intensive one-week laparoscopy training program on laparoscopic skills among postgraduate urologists. JSLS. 2008;12:1–8.
32. Udomsawaengsup S, Pattana-arun J, Tansatit T, Pungpapong SU, Navicharern P, Sirichindakul B, Nonthasoot B, Park-art R, Sriassadaporn S, Kyttayakerana K, Wongsaisuwan M, Rojanasakul A. Minimally invasive surgery training in soft cadaver (MIST-SC). J Med Assoc Thai. 2005;88:S189–94.
33. Sharma M, Horgan A. Comparison of fresh-frozen cadaver and high-fidelity virtual reality simulator as methods of laparoscopic training. World J Surg. 2012;36:1732–7.
34. Zorn KC, Gautam G, Shalhav AL, Clayman RV, Ahlering TE, Albala DM, Lee DI, Sundaram CP, Matin SF, Castle EP, Winfield HN, Gettman MT, Lee BR, Thomas R, Patel VR, Leveillee RJ, Wong C, Badlani GH, Rha KH, Eggener SE, Wiklund P, Mottrie A, Atug F, Kural AR, Joseph JV, Members of the Society of Urologic Robotic Surgeons. Training, credentialing, proctoring and medicolegal risks of robotic urological surgery: recommendations of the society of urologic robotic surgeons. J Urol. 2009;182:1126–32.
35. Macafee DA. Is there a role for mentoring in Surgical Specialty training? Med Teach. 2008;30:e55–9.
36. Hanly EJ, Miller BE, Kumar R, Hasser CJ, Coste-Maniere E, Talamini MA, Aurora AA, Schenkman NS, Marohn MR. Mentoring console improves collaboration and teaching in surgical robotics. J Laparoendosc Adv Surg Tech A. 2006;16:445–51.
37. O'Leary DP, Corrigan MA, McHugh SM, Hill AD, Redmond HP. From theater to the world wide web–a new online era for surgical education. J Surg Educ. 2012;69:483–6.

38. Knapp H, Chan K, Anaya HD, Goetz MB. Interactive internet-based clinical education: an efficient and cost-savings approach to point-of-care test training. Telemed J E Health. 2011;17:335–40.
39. Roshier AL, Foster N, Jones MA. Veterinary students' usage and perception of video teaching resources. BMC Med Educ. 2011;11:1–13.
40. McDougall EM, Corica FA, Chou DS, Abdelshehid CS, Uribe CA, Stoliar G, Sala LG, Khonsari SS, Eichel L, Boker JR, Ahlering TE, Clayman RV. Short-term impact of a robot-assisted laparoscopic prostatectomy 'mini-residency' experience on postgraduate urologists' practice patterns. Int J Med Robot. 2006;2:70–4.
41. Eliyahu S, Roguin A, Kerner A, Boulos M, Lorber A, Halabi M, Suleiman M, Nikolsky E, Rispler S, Beyar R. Patient safety and outcomes from live case demonstrations of interventional cardiology procedures. JACC Cardiovasc Interv. 2012;5:215–24.
42. Duty B, Okhunov Z, Friedlander J, Okeke Z, Smith A. Live surgical demonstrations: an old, but increasingly controversial practice. Urology. 2012;79:1185.e7–11.

Chapter 10
Teletraining in Minimal Access Surgery

Cavit Avci and Levent Avtan

Introduction

The developments in telecommunication and computer technology have made great strides, and provided considerable possibilities for education and training in Minimal Access Surgery (MAS).

In this chapter, the different applications of teletraining in MAS are described. In the first part, after an overview of telemedicine, the roles of teleconferencing, telementoring and telesurgery for teletraining in MAS are discussed. In the second part, the experiences of the coauthors are summarized.

Telemedicine

The term telemedicine has a number of definitions, but a commonly used definition proposed by The Society of American Gastrointestinal and Endoscopic Surgeons (SAGES) is: "The practice of medicine and/or teaching of the medical art, without direct physical physician-patient or physician-student interaction, via an interactive audio-video communication system employing tele-electronic devices" [1].

C. Avci, MD (✉)
General Surgery, İstanbul Medical Faculty, Istanbul University, Continuing Medical Education & Research Center, Millet Caddesi/Çapa – Şehremini, Istanbul 34390, Turkey
e-mail: cavitavci@gmail.com

L. Avtan, MD
General Surgery, İstanbul Faculty of Medicine, Istanbul University, Turgut Ozal Street, Çapa – Fatih, Istanbul, Beşiktaş 34093, Turkey
e-mail: leventavtan@gmail.com

N. Francis et al. (eds.), *Training in Minimal Access Surgery*,
DOI 10.1007/978-1-4471-6494-4_10

Today, with improvement in telecommunication and computer technology and inexpensive video-conferencing equipment, telemedicine has become easy and affordable. It is used as a means of transferring medical knowledge, and in current surgical practice can be used for training and education including the transmission of images and live video, worldwide. Telemedicine is useful and advantageous, particularly in distant learning and remote education by saving time and travel cost. It provides medical-surgical expertise to a rural area, eliminating the distance barriers by means of advanced telecommunications and information systems. The internet has an important role in the current application of telemedicine. In the last two decades, more readily available broadband internet access, which uses real-time video and information, offers the potential to increase the availability of training in minimal access surgery.

Telemedicine can be used in two ways in current practice; asynchronous or synchronous.

Asynchronous, "store and forward" is primarily used for transferring digital images (X-rays, MRIs, etc.) to a remote location. Synchronous, "real time" uses video-conferencing and patient monitoring technologies for direct care, consultation and collaboration, or a combination of the two.

Telemedicine is becoming used more in today's training of minimal access surgery with three subdivisions: Teleconference (Video conference), Telementoring and Telesurgery.

Teleconference in MAS

Teleconference has been popular in the medical environment when the asynchronous radiologic and pathologic images are sent electronically between remote hospitals in rural area to obtain a professional opinions and an exact diagnosis. In 1962, DeBakey [2] carried out international video-conferencing for the first time, with a demonstration of open-heart surgery performed in Houston, Texas, United States and transmitted overseas via satellite, allowing real time viewing of an aortic valve replacement in Geneva, Switzerland.

The use of teleconference in education and training of MAS, has become useful, efficacious and relatively easier with the improvement of technology. To get a successful teleconference under good conditions in the field of conventional and/or minimal access surgery, the transmission quality of images and sounds should be satisfactory and appropriate for the needs of surgical professionals. The International Telecommunication Union (ITU) has defined several technical standards for video-conferencing equipment: Clear regulations for sound, video, parallel video streams, and data encryption as well patient security, confidentiality, and privacy were set under those standards [3]. Four methods for data transmission during video-conferencing are available: *Integrated Services Digital Network* (*ISDN*), *satellite communication*, *Internet Protocol* (*IP*)*-based communication*, *Mobile phones* (*3G* and *4G/LTE*).

Today, almost every personal computer is able to perform basic videoconferencing at a low cost with relatively high quality due to the technologic advancements and development of network infrastructures. Currently, it can be recommended for teaching new operative techniques in MAS, especially for surgeons working in remote area and having limited possibilities for continuing education.

Telementoring in MAS

The term "surgical telementoring" is used to describe the guidance of a less experienced surgeon by an expert surgeon in a different location, using telecommunication facilities. It has an important place for training in MAS, wherein surgical techniques and technologies are constantly developing. Many active surgeons feel compelled to learn these improvements but are already busy with current practice and have little time to re-train or take sabbaticals to learn new skills necessary to carry out novel or complex procedures. Learning to perform a new laparoscopic surgical technique can be extremely challenging. The ideal approach to achieve proficiency with any new technique involves on-site observation of an experienced surgeon-mentor, followed by mentored hands-on experience of the surgeon-learner. However, it is not always feasible for a surgeon-mentor to offer on-site supervision to the surgeon-learner in his or her home institution. This is why telementoring can be a very effective solution for training in MAS. Advances in telecommunication systems and internet applications have made remote telementoring a viable alternative to on-site mentoring in selected situations.

Technical Considerations

Telementoring requires a telelink running via a limited or wide area network. A "LAN" (Local Area Network) runs within a hospital, medical university campus, building or institution, while a "WAN" (Wide Area Network) runs across the world, connecting countries, towns or buildings.

The security of the telecommunication is important. To ensure security, the network path should not allow other connections. This is a VPN ('virtual private network'), and provides a common path for video transmission. All networks now use the internet, and each individual station has a unique global address provided by the IP (internet protocol) address. Telementoring also requires a secure, highspeed internet connection with sufficient bandwidth to provide satisfactory picture quality at the mentor's location. The connection must transmit sound and vision in both directions. It has been shown that surgeons are generally able to compensate for delays (latencies) of up to 700 ms but delays above this are quite noticeable, even though telementoring has been successfully performed with greater latencies. If using an integrated services digital network (ISDN) connection, a bandwidth of 384 Kb/s (six lines) is generally needed to give sufficient picture quality for accurate interpretation by the mentor, although clinical work has been carried out using bandwidths as low as 128 Kb/s.

There are three subdivisions in using of telementoring according to the level of interaction from the mentor:

1. *Teleproctoring* (oral instructions): In the simple form, it can be as simple as verbal guidance, interactions involving audio dialogue, while watching transmitted, real-time video footage of the trainee surgeon operating.
2. *Telestration* (visual assisted mentoring): In this more complex forms, using a technology called telestration, mentor can involve indicating target areas on the local monitor screen which can be visuliased by the trainee Telestrators allow surgeons to draw a freehand sketch stream (video telestration with video tablet and pen), over the live video, which enables the mentors to convey their teaching both visually as well as verbally.
3 Teleassistance (control of the camera and remote assistance with instruments): In the last form; mentor can controlling the endoscopic or laparoscopic camera with a surgical robot such as da Vinci S surgical system to remotely assist n surgery (Intuitive Surgical, Sunnyvale, CA, USA, or taking over as the assistant by controlling retractors and instruments via a robotic arm [4].

Telesurgical Mentoring

This term was originally coined by the group at Johns Hopkins Hospital, which was one of the pioneering institutions for telementoring. One early work published by Moore et al. in 1996 described the initial clinic experience of Johns Hopkins University group (reference?). With an experienced remote surgeon successfully supervising an inexperienced surgeon 300 miles away. Mentoring was accomplished with real-time video images, two-way audio communication, a robotic arm used to control the videoendoscope, and a telestrator (Cody Sketchpad, Chryon Corp., Melville, NY) to indicate important features on the surgeon's screen [5].

Following their success of their earlier experience with telementoring they increased the distance to the remote site, while incorporating controls to a robotic arm that manipulated the laparoscope and gave access to electrocautery devices for tissue cutting or hemostasis during the telementored cases. They named this technique "telesurgical mentoring" [6].

Using a similar set-up to the group at Johns Hopkins, the first international telesurgical mentoring procedure was performed between Baltimore, USA and Innsbruck, Austria (laparoscopic adrenalectomy) and subsequently between Baltimore and Singapore (laparoscopic varicocelectomy), using three ISDN lines with a bandwidth of 384 Kb/s, and adapting for an approximate 1 s delay [7].

Ramshaw et al. Successfully telementored a rural surgeon in more than 24 cases of laparoscopic herniorrhaphy, all of which were completed successfully [8].

Surgeons on the USS Abraham Lincoln Aircraft Carrier performed five laparoscopic inguinal hernia repairs aboard the naval vessel, under telementored guidance from land-based surgeons thousand of miles away in Maryland and California. These were the first telementored laparoscopic procedures performed aboard a naval vessel and established the ability to perform long-distance intercontinental telementoring [9].

Kavoussi's group utilised the Aesop™ robot and the Socrates telestration system (Intuitive Surgical) to telementor 17 urologic operations between Baltimore, Maryland and Rome, Italy. The connections were established through 4 ISDN lines and the procedures were associated with a half second image delay between the two sites [10].

In 2003, the Vitor da Silva group from London, Ontario, Canada harnessed SOCRATES™ and AESOP™ telerobotic technology through 4 ISDN lines to successfully telementor laparoscopic nephrectomy and pyeloplasty with the mentor situated over 200 km away. Subsequently, they prospectively tested telementoring in the most technically challenging operations, such as laparoscopic radical prostatectomy and they concluded that performance of telementoring is feasible and that it is possible to teach complex operations with current technology. They have concluded that telementoring using existing communication ISDN lines is feasible and relatively inexpensive. However, its eventual adaptation in healthcare will depend on further education and an evolution in surgical thinking [11].

Rodrigues Netto Jr et al. reported in 2003 that the Johns Hopkins group successfully telementored a laparoscopic bilateral varicocelectomy and percutaneous renal access for nephro-lithotomy between Baltimore and Sao Paulo, Brazil [12].

Schlacta's group reported in 2009 that they had successfully trained less-experienced community-based general surgeons (through direct local and telementoring) to perform laparoscopic colon surgery [13]. The group concluded that telementoring could be used to teach complex operative procedures, such as laparoscopic colectomy to surgeons.

Remote Presence and Telementoring

There are few mobile wireless robots that can serve as a valuable tool for laparoscopic telementoring.

The RP-7 (RP-7*i*); In touch Health, Santa Barbara, (California) is an example of a high-end robotic remote presence system that can be controlled by a portable personal computer linked via an internet connection. Its dimensions are 165 cm in height and 63 cm × 76 cm at its base, comparable in size to that of an average human. The head of the robot is equipped with two advanced digital cameras, audio microphone and sophisticated engineering allows a real-time, two-way audio-video link. In addition the robot is highly manoeuvrable and allows a wide range of motions, *e.g.*, panning and tilting [14].

Antonio Marttos et al. reported in 2012 assessed the use of a telepresence robot (VISITOR1™) in the operating room in 50 surgical cases [15]. The Karl

Storz-InTouch VISITOR1™ system is an intra-operative, spring arm-mounted communications platform comprising a control station and a robot. The control station and robot are linked via the internet over a secure broadband connection. Through the control station, either installed on a laptop or desktop computer, a remote physician can gain access to the operating room from home or office. The system communicates bi-directionally using TCP and/or UDP, and requires outbound HTTP access to connect to the In Touch Health servers. The VISITOR1™ system incorporates encryption methodology utilizing a combination of RSA public/private key and 128-bit AES symmetric encryption.

Sereno et al. described a successful experiment using the previous version of the remote presence robot the RP-6 (predecessor to the RP-7) [16]. They have used two mentoring methods; (1) "active onsite mentoring" and (2) "passive onsite mentoring". The noted that hands-on training courses with local mentoring were excellent educational tools in laparoscopic surgery; however, the need for the physical presence of specialized instructors represented a limitation because of costs, time, and geographic constraints. Remote robotic telementoring using a wireless video-conferencing mobile robot could represent an alternative to local instruction.

Bogen et al. conducted several successful pilot experiments at their department with a low cost telementoring prototype, based on a home personal computer and a tablet, with telementoring performed over the internet [17]. Their software and hardware solution allowed them to capture the laparoscopic image directly from the laparoscopic camera and perform several different image manipulations in real time. The software provided a secure platform that follows and complies with The Health Insurance Portability and Accountability Act of 1996 Privacy, Security and Breach Notification Rules and regulations (HIPAA). They stated that this technique is transferable and reproducible to all laparoscopic disciplines *e.g.*, robotic surgery and endoscopy. So far they conducted successful episodes of telementoring in colorectal surgery (abdomino-perineal resection), in urological surgery (adrenalectomy, nephropexy and robotic assisted laparoscopic prostatectomy) [17].

Telesurgery

Telesurgery involves a surgical procedure with the surgeon being situated remotely from the patient. The history of telesurgery dates back to the first commercial application in laparoscopy.

When AESOP™ (The Automated Endoscopic System for Optimal Positioning) was initially introduced and used solely to guide the laparoscope, the surgeon controlled the robotic arm either manually or remotely with hand or foot switches. Later versions were modified and equipped with voice controls. Although their use has been associated with 'telementoring procedures', its development gave way to the complex three armed robotic technology that integrated instrument manipulating arms as well. The manufacturer of the AESOP™, Computer Motion Inc., later introduced the three armed ZEUS™ robotic system onto the market in 1998. Concurrently, Intuitive Surgical (Sunnyvale, California) released yet another 3-arm surgical robot, the da Vinci, developed from technology designed by the The National Aeronautics and Space Administration (NASA). With the introduction of the Zeus® and Da Vinci® robots (Intuitive Surgical, Mountain View, CA) the possibility of true telesurgery arrived [18].

The First Telesurgical Trans-Atlantic Robotic Operation

In 2001, Marescaux et al. expanded this type of surgery surgery by performing a trans-Atlantic robotic assisted cholecystectomy (Lindbergh procedure) using the Zeus® robot [19]. The surgeon and console were located in New York, and the patient and effector arms were in Strasbourg, France. Asynchronous transfer mode (ATM) technology was used to establish connections via high-speed terrestrial fibre-optic networks with a bandwidth of 10 Mb/s. These connections were reserved exclusively for the procedure that ran a round-trip distance of 14,000 km. Although there was a lag time of 155 ms, the laparoscopic cholecystectomy was completed without incident in 54 min. It should be noted that although audiovisual interactions and robotic arm movements were performed through the trans-Atlantic connections, the application of 'electrocautery' to dissect the gall bladder, placement of clips, introduction of the ports, and closure of port-sites had to be performed by the assistants in the remote operating room. Laparoscopic cholecystectomy is a relatively simple laparoscopic procedure and was feasible to complete the operation safely by the remote surgeons. Although the cost of this solitary operation was astronomical, it demonstrated that 'real world' long-distance telesurgery was feasible, and if the lag time could be limited to <155 ms, surgeons could perform operative procedures from their home base, even if the patient was on a battlefield or in the far reaches of space.

Currently, the large majority of published literature on robotic-assisted surgery, has employed the use of the da Vinci system, because today it is the only commercially available surgical robotic system.

Telemedicine

Despite the advantages associated with telementoring and telesurgery, there are a number of significant technical and ethical issues.

Cost Limitations and Latency

Telementoring requires a secure high-speed connection with sufficient bandwidth to provide high quality video and audio at both the mentor and trainee stations. One of the disadvantages is the initial set-up cost, the costs of consumables and maintenance. The cost of buying a telecommunication system and installing cabling for a hard-wired connection is relatively high, and leased lines from telecommunications companies will eventually exceed this initial outlay. The reliability of the link itself is also an issue, as it could be potentially disastrous to lose the connection at a critical stage during an operation. Another problem is that telementoring requires an optimal latency (the amount of time it takes a packet to travel from source to destination) of, ideally, no more than 700 ms; high latency results in extreme degradation of the mentor's view of the procedure and can been a major set-back in a live videoconferencing session.

Ethical and Medico-Legal Considerations

When a surgeon in one location operates a patient in another remote location, different institution or country, several major ethical and medico-legal issues arise. Surgical insurance policies for individual surgeons or institutions are usually specific to a country or even a region or state. Additionally, during a telementored surgical procedure the primary surgeon, at the remote operating theatre, has primary medical authority and is the sole responsible surgeon ultimately liable for malpractice during the surgery. The premise is that the mentoring surgeon is providing only recommendations and a professional opinion. For now, there are no definitive answers for some of the medico-legal issues: who assumes the primary medicolegal responsibility, the remote surgeon or the experienced mentor surgeon based from afar? What organisation, society or individual decides who is credentialed to be a mentor? What happens if the telecommunication system fails? If these problems are resolved, perhaps by the direction of an international agency, telemedicine will be able to realise its full potential.

Experiences of Teleconference and Telementoring in MAS

Teleconferencing During MAS Courses

In recent years, we have had some experience of tele-education on minimal access surgery in Istanbul University (IU), which is the initiator for videoscopic surgery and also distance education by the way of telemedicine in Turkey. The Continuous Medical Education and Research Centre of Istanbul University (ISTEM) is the centre, which conducts many educational activities and currently works in telemedicine, teleconferencing and telementoring. The regular training courses in minimal access and videoscopic (laparoscopic, endoscopic) surgery have been organised by ISTEM since 1991, in close collaboration with the Turkish Association for Endoscopic Laparoscopic Surgery (ELCD). We have trained over a thousand surgeons in MAS and awarded a certificate recognized by the European Association of Endoscopic Surgery (EAES) over 20 years. Surgical operations performed during the laparoscopic courses are transmitted from the operating room to our meeting room by our tele-conferencing system. Thus, all trainees in the meeting room can see live surgery in real time and have an interactive discussion with the operating surgeon. Sometimes, we broadcast this transmission via the internet for remote surgeons who register to receive this tele-conference.

Tele-conferencing in Residency Programme

We use also teleconferencing to exchange knowledge and expertise in various disciplines, between the two Medical schools of Istanbul University that are 7 km apart. Some weekly regular staff meetings or occasional scientific sessions for the residents are conducted by tele-conference. The audio-video presentations and discussions happen interactively and in real time. We also use tele-conferencing to interact with other affiliated teaching hospitals in Istanbul, or in different areas of Turkey.

International Tele-conferencing Programme

Having sufficient experience with tele-conferencing in Turkey, we decided to expand internationally. A multi-national project was planned. The main objective was to promote an international exchange of knowledge about video-scopic surgery and establish a surgical network with high-quality moving images over broadband internet access. With this objective, we created the web-telesurgery platform in 2009. It is a free online platform for training, education and communication of surgery, especially videoscopic surgery. It has been created by the ISTEM team in Istanbul and is managed by an international educational and evaluation board" (where is the other quotation mark?). Its main objective is to expand medico-surgical knowledge, in collaboration with the major scientific associations and centres of excellence in Europe. A low-bandwidth internet-based system was selected, assuring the online tele-transmission of an optimal quality of video-audio, as well as the required interactivity for learning.

Networks

We are connecting the operating rooms and conference room via hospital network which will be connected to our Portable Wireless Live Video/Audio Transmission System (IMD), or to our personal computer containing special converting software. We usually use Adobe Flash Media Live Decoder to convert directly the digital video signals to IP format. We sometimes use the DVTS (Digital Video Transport System) that is a kind of software used mainly by the Asia Pacific Telemedicine Group for sending and receiving digital video streams through the internet [20]. It is an open source freeware that can be downloaded from the web site. We have

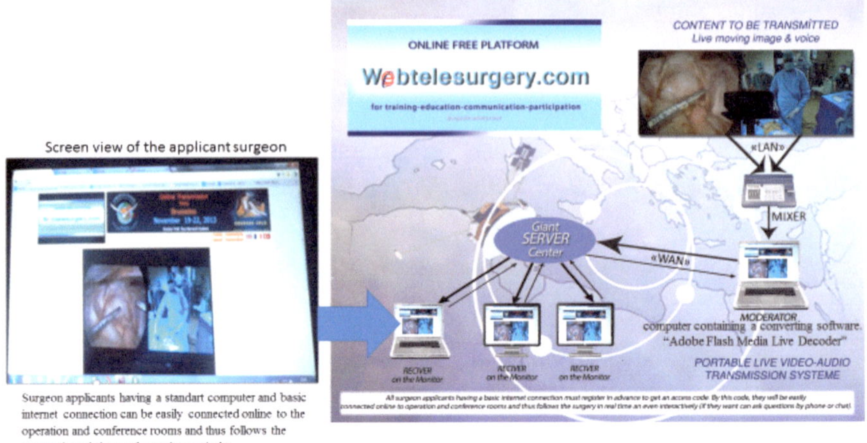

Fig. 10.1 The Network Configuration. Online broadcasting of a videoscopic courses with "webtelesurgery.com"

recently focussed on Video, that is another new videoconferencing system [21]. The audio-visual content is sent via a dedicated broadband internet connection, minimum 1 or 2 Megabits per second, to our main server, and then distributed to individual receivers (Fig. 10.1). Surgeons having a standard computer and basic internet connection must register in advance to get an access code that we provide. With this code, they will be easily connected online to the operation and conference rooms and thus follow the surgery in real time and even interactively by phone.

Low-bandwidth internet-based telemedicine is effective and inexpensive. Surgeons living in remote areas, distant countries and especially those with limited resources, can follow the videoscopic courses, meetings and live surgeries organized by experienced centres, on their computer screen, in real-time and interactively.

Convention with ESLS in Brussels and Cooperation with MMESA

The European School of Laparoscopic Surgery (ESLS) at the Saint-Pierre University Hospital in Brussels is one of the oldest and famous schools of laparoscopic surgery in Europe. ESLS in Brussels and ISTEM & ELCD in Istanbul have created a convention on tele-training and tele-teaching using the Webtelesurgery platform. With this convention, we have established a partnership with MMESA (Mediterranean and Middle-eastern Endoscopic Surgery Association) to broadcast courses, congresses or specific educational training sessions about MAS, organized by ourselves and/or by famous teams in Europe and the Middle East. MMESA includes 36 Countries around the Mediterranean Sea and the Middle East. It is an open association and other countries from Africa, the Black Sea region or Central Asia have also joined this project.

The ESLS regularly organizes 15–17 advanced laparoscopic courses (general, bariatric, colorectal, hernia repair, trans-oral foregut and nursing) every year in St. Pierre University Hospital in Brussels. The group of ISTEM-ELCD also organize courses and educational meetings in Istanbul. For 5 years, we have transmitted some of these courses and activities, via the webtelesurgery platform to the world, especially to the MMESA countries. These transmissions are always free of charge and many surgeons, especially from the developing countries can be connected very easily and at a very low cost, needing only a computer and simple internet connection. Earlier technical difficulties with the sound and the quality of the picture have been overcome.

Live Broadcasting of Meetings and Congresses

In recent years, thanks to our portable teleconferencing system, we conducted live broadcasts of a f meetings and conferences from France, to the French-speaking countries of North Africa. Meeting "Mesh" in 1998, 99 and 2001, organized in Paris by the French Laparoscopic Surgery Society (SFCL) team were sent via Internet using our teleconferencing system, to Maghreb countries. Many surgeons in Algeria, Tunisia and Morocco are connected and supported by distance interactively (question-response by phone/Skype) in this meeting

In 2008 and 2009, the Video Forum in Digestive Surgery, organized by the University of Toulouse in France, was transmitted to francophone countries. The two Congresses of Coelio Surgery Lyon, which took place in Lyon, France, in 2011.

Broadcasting of Videoscopic Surgery Courses Between Turkey and Azerbaijan

Live bariatric surgery courses were organized by the ELCD team in İstanbul University Hospital and broadcast through the internet to the Medical University of Azerbaijan, Baku in 2014 (Fig. 10.2). Twenty two Turkish surgeons on site in the meeting room of ISTEM in Istanbul and more than a hundred Azeri surgeons participated online in Baku. The audio-visual connection between the operating room and the conference room of ISTEM in Istanbul was made by the hospital's intranet (LAN). Re-transmission of the course content (live operations and discussions) was carried out via the internet in real time using our teleconference system of "webtelesugery.com". The return of video and audio from Baku to Istanbul was through

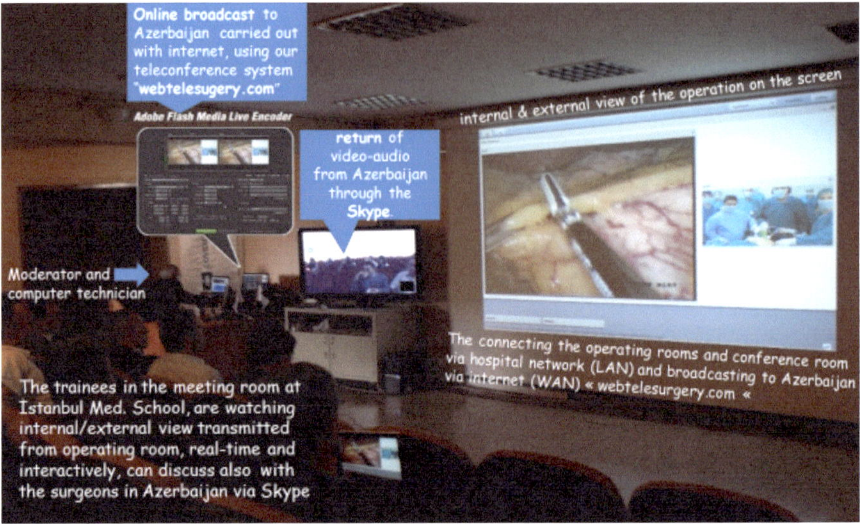

Fig. 10.2 Broadcasting of videoscopic surgery courses between Turkey and Azerbaijan

Skype. The quality of picture and sound was satisfactory in spite of the relatively long time delay. This experience of telemedicine between Istanbul and Baku was encouraging for us to continue collaboration through telemedicine with the Azerbaijan and subsequently with other Turkish-speaking countries.

Our Experience of Local and Remote Telementoring in MAS

We use the telementoring in different ways, depending on the near (Local telementoring in the residency programme) or distant location (Remote telementoring in the national programme). The installation, preparation and tele-connection are slightly different.

Local Telementoring/Telestration in Residency Programme

We regularly use the local telementoring in our hospital to train our residents and young surgeons. Of course, direct (on site) mentoring in operating room for less experienced surgeons is better, but in current practice, it is still not possible, due the very busy schedule and other obligations of a university professor. For this reason, telementoring in university and non-academic educational hospitals is efficacious and recommended, as a complementary method for residency training in surgery. When we are not available to assist the less experienced resident in operating room, we can connect online from our office, see the outcome of surgery and if necessary

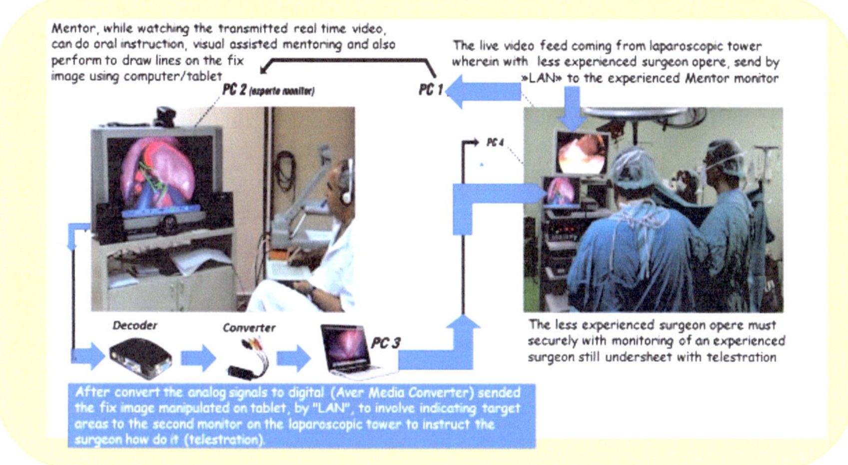

Fig. 10.3 The schema of the telementoring/telestration in our hospital to train our residents

can help him/her with telementoring or telestration. Teleconnection is made relatively easily and effectively with the hospital intranet (LAN). This easy and low cost telementoring prototype is based on a standard personal computer with a media player (Aver Media Player card), a free software encoder programme (Adobe Flash Media Live Encoder 3) and a tablet (Fig. 10.3).

In the operating room, all necessary video-conferencing equipment must be tested to avoid any malfunction during telementoring. It is better that the mentor and the operating surgeon wear a headset and microphone connected to an audio-visual mixer console,to reduce background noise and enhance voice clarity. An S-video connection is made between the laparoscopic tower and a computer in the operating room. The audio-visual content passes from the computer by intranet to the mentor's personal computer to which a tablet is also connected. The mentor surgeon in his office, while watching the transmitted real time video of operation on the screen, can easily give oral instruction or visual-assisted mentoring with the cursor of the computer mouse or with a tablet pen. He can also realise the telestration, using the tablet as a tool to enhance his verbal instructions. In a delicate stage of the operation the mentor can use the tablet's pen to draw on a still image and send this image to a second monitor on the laparoscopic tower to guide the trainee surgeon during the operation. The analogue images from the monitor of the laparoscopic tower, or possibly from an external view camera is converted to digital images on the computers.

In the Istanbul Medical School Hospital, telementoring has become a complementary way to train our residents in general surgery, as well as other surgical disciplines, especially for videoscopic surgery (endoscopic laparoscopic, thoracoscopic, arthroscopic …). On the other hand, in the Continuing Medical Education (CME) programme of our university we also use remote telementoring for distance learning.

Remote Telementoring in National Programme

We sometimes carry out remote telementoring for surgeons participating in our regular videoscopic surgery courses for trainees requesting help for their first operation with the technique that have seen during a course. If he/she does not have a locally experienced colleague available to mentor the technique, we suggest a remote telementoring.

We use also remote telementoring to assist an inexperienced surgeon/trainee in rural areas, particularly for the introduction of new techniques to young surgeons when a local mentor surgeon is rarely available. The ELCD has more then 1200 members. When a distant member needs help to learn a new technique or needs help with a difficult case or consultation in an emergency situation, an experienced mentor belonging to the ELCD educational/training committee will assist by telementoring if the remote surgeon possesses the necessary means to connect.

Summary

Telemedicine is useful and advantageous, particularly in distance-learning and remote education by saving time and travel costs. The advanced telecommunications and information systems, especially broadband internet access, which uses real-time video and information offers the potential to increase the availability of training in minimal access surgery.

The use of teleconference in education and training of MAS, has become easier with the improvement of appropriate technology. Today, all surgeons, especially those in rural areas can enjoy videoconferences organized by the groups or centres of excellence disseminated via the internet. Having a personal computer and standard internet access is usually enough.

Telesurgery is an advanced stage of telementoring that is currently identified with surgical robots. Nowadays robot assisted telesurgery is under utilised due to the current technical limitations but, it has a potential role in assisting telemonitoring and remote training in future.

References

1. Guidelines for the Surgical Practice of Telemedicine. This statement was reviewed and approved by the Board of Governors of the Society of American Gastrointestinal and Endoscopic Surgeons (SAGES) on Oct 2010. publications@sages.org.
2. Augestad KM, Lindsetmo RO. Overcoming distance: videoconferencing as a clinical and educational tool among surgeons. World J Surg 2009;33:1356–65 [PMID: 19384459; doi:10.1007/s00268-009-0036-0].
3. ITU: Committed to connecting the world [Internet]. itu.int[cited 2013 Feb 26]. Available from: URL: http://www.itu.int/en/pages/default.aspx.

4. Challacombe B, et al. Technology Insight: telementoring and telesurgery in urology. Nat Clin Pract Urol. 2006;3(11):611–7.
5. Moore RG, Adams JB, Partin AW, Docimo SG, Kavoussi LR. Telementoring of laparoscopic procedures: initial clinical experience. Surg Endosc. 1996;10(2):107–10.
6. Schulam PG, et al. Telesurgical mentoring. Initialclinical experience. Surg Endosc. 1997;11:1001–5.
7. Lee BR, et al. International surgical telementoring: our initial experience. Stud HealthTechnol Inform. 1998;50:41–7.
8. Ranshaw B, Tucker J, Duncan T. Laparoscopic herniorrhaphy: a review of 900 cases. Surg Endosc. 1996;10:255.
9. Cubano M, Poulose BK, Talamini MA, Stewart R, Antosek LE, Lentz R, et al. Long distance telementoring. A novel tool for laparoscopy aboard the USS Abraham Lincoln. Surg Endosc. 1999;13(7):673–8.
10. Micali S, Virgili G, Vannozzi E, Grassi N, Jarrett TW, Bauer JJ, Kavoussi LR. Feasibility of telementoring between Baltimore (USA) and Rome (Italy): the first five cases. J Endourol. 2000;14(6):493–6.
11. Vitor da Silva, Telementoring and telesurgery: future or fiction? Source: Robot surgery, Book edited by: Seung Hyuk Baik, ISBN 978-953-7619-77-0, p. 172, January 2010, INTECH, Croatia, downloaded from SCIYO.COM.
12. Rodrigues Netto Jr N, et al. Telementoring between Brazil and the United States: initial experience. J Endourol. 2003;17:217–20.
13. Schlachta CM, Lefebvre KL, Sorsdahl AK, Jayaraman S. Mentoring and telementoring leads to effective incorporation of laparoscopic colon surgery. Surg Endosc. 2009;24(4):841–44.
14. RP-7 Remote Presence System, INTOUCH HEALT, Santa Barbara, California. 805.562.8686. www.intouchhealth.com.
15. Marttos et al. Surgical telepresence the usability of a robotic communication platform. World J Emerg Surg. 2012;7(Suppl 1):S11. http://www.wjes.org/content/7/S1/S11.
16. Sereno S, Mutter D, Dallemagne B, Smith CD, Marescaux J. Telementoring for minimally invasive surgical training bywireless robot. Surg Innov. 2007;14:184–91 [PMID: 17928617. doi:10.1177/1553350607308369].
17. Bogen EM, Augestad KM, Patel HRH, Lindsetmo RO. Telementoringin education of laparoscopic surgeons: an emerging technology. World J Gastrointest Endosc. 2014;6(5):148–55.
18. Challacombe BJ, et al. Trans oceanic telerobotic surgery. BJU Int. 2003;92:678–80.
19. Marescaux J, Leroy J, Gagner M, Rubino F, Mutter D, Vix M, et al. Transatlantic robot-assisted telesurgery. Nature. 2001;413(6854):379–80.
20. Shimizu S, Nakashima N, Okamura K, Tanaka M. One hundred case studies of Asia-Pasific telemedicine using a digital video transport systeme over a research and education network. Telemed J E Health. 2009;15:112–7.
21. Cao Duc Minh, Shuji Shimizu, et al. Emerging technologies for telemedicine. Korean J Radiol. 2012;13(Suppl 1):S21–S30.

Chapter 11
Assessment and Accreditation in MAS

Howard Champion and Abe Fingerhut

Introduction

More than two decades ago, the appeal of minimal access surgery (MAS), with its smaller footprint on the body and faster recovery times, created a demand for more procedures to be done laparoscopically [1]. Accreditation Council for Graduate Medical Education (ACGME) data indicate that between 1997 and 2010, the number of basic and advanced laparoscopic procedures (appendectomies, cholecystectomies, hernia repairs, and colectomies) performed by graduating surgical residents increased by an average of approximately one-third [2]. This trend was accompanied by an almost 45 % average decrease in performance of these procedures using open surgery [2].

The proliferation of MAS in the mid-1990s was accompanied by media attention on surgical errors in general [3], largely precipitated by a 1995 case in Florida in which a surgeon amputated the wrong leg [4]. Also at that time, a decade of pediatric heart surgery at the Bristol Royal Infirmary, England, was coming to a close that would be the subject of a widely publicized inquiry because of an excessively high death rate [5]. In 2000, the Institute of Medicine published its *To Err is Human* report [6], which focused attention on the epidemic of fatal medical errors in the United States, and thus on the need for ways to improve quality of care and reduce risk to patients. Better training and objective assessment were put forth as imperatives, and,

H. Champion, FRCS (Ed, ENG) FACS
Department of Surgery, Uniformed Services
University of the Health Sciences, Maryland, USA

A. Fingerhut, MD, DSC (Hon), FACS (✉)
Section for Surgical Research (Prof Uranues), Department of Surgery,
Medical University of Graz, Auenbruggerplatz 29, 8036 Graz, Austria

First Department of Surgery (Prof Leandros), University of Athens,
Hippokration University Hospital, Athens, Greece
e-mail: abefingerhut@aol.com

N. Francis et al. (eds.), *Training in Minimal Access Surgery*,
DOI 10.1007/978-1-4471-6494-4_11

by extension, ceasing to use live patients during trainee learning. Specifically, assessment of competency was suggested at four points along a career trajectory, *i.e.*, entering practice, maintenance of competency, reentering practice, and after a disciplinary action [7]. State regulation was recommended to ensure that clinicians establish and prove their ability to perform all requisite technical and non-technical skills.

The technical differences between MAS and open surgery have led to wide recognition of the specific challenges associated with attainment of proficiency in MAS. These include eye-hand co-ordination in a 3-D environment when visual orientation is in 2-D. As was made clear in several studies of errors in laparoscopic cholecystectomy in the mid-1990s [8–10], MAS has a learning curve caused, at least in part, by "inadequate training in the skills necessary to overcome the psychomotor hurdles imposed by this new technology." [3] Kumar & Gill [11] noted that "laparoscopic skills are not an innate behavior and can be learned only with the aid of hands-on training. "Using the example of laparoscopic nephrectomy, they documented how even surgeons who are experienced in the open technique have high initial MAS complication rates, which then decrease with subsequent repetitions. In an international multicenter trial of 1844 laparoscopic prostatectomies performed by 51 surgeons, Secin et al. [12] found that the learning curve plateaued at 200–250 cases. Notably, the learning curve was not influenced at all by experience with the open technique, which led the authors to conclude that "specifically laparoscopic training and experience" are needed to reach the desired level of proficiency [13].

"The technical skills needed for laparoscopic surgery are fundamentally different from those for traditional open surgery.... It is evident... that laparoscopy is associated with a longer operation time and a higher rate of surgical complications during the learning curve of the surgeons" [13].

Why the Need for Assessment?

There are a variety of ways of teaching and assessing basic MAS skills. Today, these almost exclusively involve simulators, which range from physical systems such as the McGill Inanimate System for Training and Evaluation of Laparoscopic Skills (MISTELS) used in the Fundamentals of Laparoscopic Surgery (FLS) program [15], to virtual reality (VR) simulation. Although, as noted by Stefanides et al. [16], "it is still unclear which simulators should be used in which context of training and with what type of learner," Simulation-based training of any kind, not just in medicine, promotes standardization of procedures, allows repetitive practice until proficiency is attained, and provides trainees with performance feedback. VR simulation has been demonstrated to be effective in improving MAS performance. In a 2002 randomized, double-blinded study, VR surgical simulation significantly improved residents' performance of laparoscopic cholecystectomy [17]. In another example, VR simulator training was associated with an increase in novice trainees' laparoscopic salpingectomy skills from beginner- to intermediate-level, with a decrease in operative time from 24 to 12 min [8]. Recent studies bolster these findings that skills learned on a VR simulator transfer to higher levels of skill in the OR [18, 19].

"Most general surgery residencies include basic laparoscopic procedures within their residency case repertoire, including diagnostic laparoscopy, laparoscopic cholecystectomy, and laparoscopic appendectomy. The experience with more advanced laparoscopic cases such as antireflux surgery, inguinal and ventral herniorrhaphy, solid organ surgery, colorectal surgery, gastric and intestinal resections, and donor nephrectomy is more variable" [14].

Obviously, acquiring advanced MAS skills is more challenging than mastering the basics, and is largely dependent upon repetitive practice [20]. Residents have often lacked opportunities to practice advanced MAS procedures, however, in part due to insufficient case volume. Laparoscopic fellowships have begun to make headway in solving this problem [21].

Perhaps the most effective avenue for attaining proficiency in advanced MAS techniques is simulation-based training. The primary advantage is that it allows consequence-free practice to proficiency, or creation of what Gallagher et al. termed the "pre-trained novice." [22] This is especially important in disciplines such as MAS, where the axiom of "see one, do one, teach one" is inverted. Learning laparoscopic skills begins with "do one" because only hands-on practice, not observation, effectively imparts the necessary skills [23–26]. Proficiency in laparoscopic knot tying, for example, was only gained via repeated practice in an evaluation of structured and quantitative methods for teaching this skill [27]. The truism, "practice makes perfect" has been proven repeatedly in laparoscopy and in other medical/surgical areas, although, as noted by expertise researcher K. Anders Ericsson, the practice must be deliberate practice if expertise is to be attained and maintained [28–30].

The use of innovative simulator devices that train surgical tasks and basic skills through repetitive, proctored challenges may lead to better detection and analysis of potential surgical errors. Error reduction and surgical expertise could be achieved through a simulator-based curriculum that assesses skill acquisition and attainment through objective measurements. With exposure to such a curriculum, surgical trainees may be able to achieve a considerable level of expertise, allowing for higher quality healthcare provision during their residency training and beyond [20].

As is the case for surgical training in general, MAS training has room for increased standardization, access, and assessment. A survey sent to US surgery program directors (with a 38 % response rate, N=95) yielded disparate results (*e.g.*, only half of the programs had dedicated MAS rotations), leading the authors to conclude that more opportunities for MAS training are needed [31].

What Constitutes Assessment?

Components of Assessment

According to the Director of Research, Center for Advanced Medical Learning and Simulation (CAMLS), University of South Florida (Janis Cannon-Bowers, PhD, personal communications, August 16, 2012), assessment of surgical training

Table 11.1 Modified hierarchy of surgical training effectiveness

Assessment components	Determinants of training effectiveness
Pre-training assessment	Establish whether trainees can be reasonably expected to benefit from the training Indicates whether or not remediation should occur prior to training.
Reactions	Determine whether trainees find the training enjoyable Determine whether trainees believe that the training has value to their development Determine whether trainees display high degrees of self-efficacy
Motivation	Determine whether the system has intrinsic motivational value
Learning	Determine whether appropriate learning has occurred
Training performance (behavior)	Determine whether appropriate skills have been mastered and can be demonstrated, including psychomotor skills, psychomotor fluency, judgment/decision making, stress inoculation
Transfer of Training	Determine whether learning in training has desired effect on real world performance using a near transfer paradigm
Results	Determine whether the investment in training was justified in terms of achieved outcomes (*i.e.*, elimination or drastic reduction of live tissue use)

effectiveness can be accomplished using a modified version of Kirkpatrick's 1976 hierarchy [32] (reaction, learning, behavior, results). This model, used extensively throughout industry and the military, has the following components: pre-training assessment, reactions/motivation, learning, training behavior, transfer of training, and organizational results (Table 11.1).

Pre-training Assessment

Pre-training assessment determines whether students have the cognitive or affective prerequisites for training, such as aptitudes (cognitive and physical ability), prerequisites (prior knowledge and experience), and attitudes (motivation for and instrumentality of training). This type of assessment can indicate the need for remedial (pre-training) training, or for tailoring the training to specific needs (*e.g.*, by starting with less challenging scenarios).

Reactions/Motivation

Reactions/motivation speaks to students' beliefs about the value or utility of the training, and is a predictor of performance and transfer of training, as is self-efficacy, or confidence in one's abilities. Self-efficacy can be measured using self-efficacy scales [33], which quantify confidence along an ascending scale (from 0 – cannot do, to 100 – can almost certainly do) [34].

Learning and Training Behavior

Learning reflects cognitive change, and is typically assessed via recognition or recall tests. When dealing with complex higher-order skills (*e.g.*, MAS), these are not sufficient to capture whether appropriate learning has occurred. Rather, declarative and procedural knowledge assessments are needed to ensure that a sufficient knowledge base to support higher-order performance is established in trainees. Training behavior, or demonstration of skill mastery, is more challenging to measure than learning because it usually involves a concrete demonstration, which is not amenable to written tests. In MAS, critical psychomotor skills can be assessed using metrics obtained from digital or sensor technologies embedded in simulations. Psychomotor fluency or automaticity can also be assessed with instrumented simulations and video recording of performance. Assessment of judgment/decision-making can be accomplished by presenting students with case scenarios, in which they are required to rapidly recognize a situation and take appropriate action under a variety of stressful conditions (*e.g.*, requiring them to perform at faster than normal speeds). These methods have been developed in military medical simulation environments.

Transfer of Training

Transfer of newly learned material to the operational environment is a complex phenomenon that encompasses a variety of factors [35]. A consistent finding from past work indicates that even when trainees have mastered the competencies for effective performance, it does not necessarily mean they will use those skills in practice. These findings complicate the assessment of transfer because it is often not clear why trainees fail to transfer what they learned (*i.e.*, it could be because the training was inadequate or due to an environmental factor). One way to make transfer of training more likely is to create a highly realistic, authentic (*e.g.*, VR) environment in which to help trainees gain self-efficacy.

Organizational Results

The final level in Kirkpatrick's hierarchy involves determining whether the organization's goals (*e.g.*, safety, productivity, reduced costs, reduction of errors, quality/quantity of performance, profit, job satisfaction, personal growth) were served by the training. An organizational goal of the US military, for example, is to reduce the use of live animals used in medical training. An organizational goal shared by all is improved patient safety, which is facilitated by improved training.

Formative and Summative Assessment

Training and assessment are often viewed as activities that should be integrated if either is to be effective. In their paper on assessment of clinical competence, Wass et al. [36] discuss the need for both formative and summative assessment in medical education. In formative assessments, students gain knowledge from tests and are given immediate feedback that they can use to correct their mistakes and refine their knowledge and skills. Summative assessments judge student performance for the purpose of evaluating clinical competence, and necessarily include definitions of failure and success. Wass and colleagues stressed the importance of using both types of assessment; "if assessment focuses only on certification and exclusion," they assert, "the all important influence on the learning process will be lost" [36].

This sentiment is echoed by Handfield-Jones et al. [37], who described formative assessment as a way to enhance the learning process and summative assessment as tool to use when intermediate or target endpoints have been identified [38]. Frequent assessments, they maintain, provide students with many points at which they can correct and enhance their performance, and advocate the use of both formative and summative assessments. "If a resident does not receive or accurately process faculty formative or summative evaluations," state Peyre et al., "then they [*sic*] can develop an inaccurate perception of their [*sic*] abilities" (more on self-assessment below) [39].

Curriculum-Based Context for Assessment

Surgical training development ideally begins with definition of a set of desired outcome measures that describe what the learner should be able to accomplish upon completion of the course. Next, each procedural step and assessment mechanism should be defined (see list below). Developing competency benchmarks for each outcome measure is a critical step in ensuring that learners attain a minimum level of competency based upon established, quantifiable definitions of success. These benchmarks can be objectively defined as follows:

- Have experts in the procedure perform the tasks until their learning curves plateau
- Determine the mean and standard deviation of the average score of the experts
- Define the benchmark for novices as one standard deviation below the expert mean
- Define the benchmark for experienced practitioners as the expert mean
- Define competence as scoring at or above the benchmark on two consecutive trials

Surgical Course Development Steps

1. *Define task or procedure to be taught*

2. *Deconstruct task into the sequence of individual steps to be performed*
3. *Analyze each step to ensure that it is needed and accurately defined*
4. *Define common errors for each task or step with a potentially serious error*
5. *Define metrics for each task and error; quantify using a measurement such as time or location along a scale*
6. *If using a scale, define all points along the scale accurately and with high inter-rater reliability*
7. *Define an assessment tool for each task and error (quantify as above)*

Surgical training necessarily consists of both cognitive and technical components. As suggested above, effectiveness of cognitive training can be assessed by (1) an initial pretest of requisite principles; (2) didactic instruction, including error identification; and (3) a post-test. Ideally, a perfect score should be attained on the post-test before the technical/psychomotor skills training portion begins; this enables errors made during the skills component to be attributable to the need for more practice rather than for rehashing of principles.

Effectiveness of the skills component should also begin with a pretest, then an initial run-through of the task by the learner, followed by as many repetitions of the task as needed until the agreed-upon level of competency is attained. In the event that training to competency is not possible, a post-test can be given when the learner has completed a predetermined number of trials to ascertain if he or she has successfully attained the desired skills.

Technical Skills Assessment in MAS

As discussed above, the technical skills needed for performing MAS are unique to MAS. In a 2002 study, Payandeh et al. explored the definition of metrics for assessing laparoscopic surgical skills [40]. In one study, novice and expert surgical residents were videotaped while performing four MAS tasks (suturing, tying knots [41], cutting suture, and dissecting tissue) in an animal lab, and their performance was analyzed [42]. Five basic motions were identified, *i.e.*, (1) reach and orient, (2) grasp and hold/cut, (3) push, (4) pull, and (5) release. Time duration to complete these tasks was used to isolate and compare subtasks, *e.g.*, dissecting tissue had the two subtasks of pulling tissue taut and snipping tissue. From this analysis, the time to complete the pull taut tissue subtask emerged as an important differentiator between novice and expert performance. A similar conclusion was reached when time to complete the seven subtasks of the suture task (position needle, bite tissue, pull needle through tissue, reposition, re-bite tissue, re-pull needle, and pull suture through) was analyzed. "Hence, any training system," the authors concluded, "should have components that train novices in these subtasks with the aim of reducing the time taken during the subtasks."

In addition to time being a key metric for MAS assessment, hand-eye coordination tasks (dexterity) were shown to be important in MAS training. Dexterity was measured by total deviation of the path from the nominal trajectory, force profile on the object created by the novice, and total number of contact discontinuities created when tracing the nominal path.

"Progress in the design of simulators for the training of laparoscopic surgical skills will require three parallel approaches: increasingly realistic simulations of surgical environments, the study of human interactivity in real-time systems with minimal lag [43], *and content based on empirical studies of surgeons' cognitive processes and visuomotor skills"* [44].

In Liang & Shi's evaluation of a virtual surgery training system (not specific to MAS), three categories of surgical skill evaluation criteria emerged: (1) efficiency, (2) safety, and (3) quality. Efficiency refers to the metrics of time to completion and redundancy of movement, safety refers to the ability to avoid "unwanted collisions" between instruments and anatomy, and quality refers to measurement of trainee performance relative to standards of success and failure [45].

Recent studies have explored the metric of force (mean, maximum, and overall magnitude) on tissue, because excessive force is a known error associated with MAS [46–48].

Learning from Mistakes

Another important factor in learning is identifying and remedying errors. As has been noted by others [49], errors may stem from failures of perception [50], knowledge, decision-making, and execution. A common serious error in MAS is injury of the bile duct during laparoscopic cholecystectomy [51], where perception errors in identifying the cystic and common ducts have caused lethal errors [52, 53]. Medical errors, as touched on briefly above, have been a worldwide problem of epidemic proportions. As for the subset that is surgical errors, more than half are due to technical mistakes [54]. The literature overwhelmingly concludes that as many as half of all surgical adverse events are preventable [55–61].

The ability of simulation-based training to reduce MAS errors has been known for some time. In 2002, a study by Seymour et al. [17] showed that, compared to controls, residents trained on a virtual reality (VR) laparoscopic cholecystectomy simulator performed gallbladder dissection 29 % faster, were nine times less likely to transiently falter (0.25 *vs*. 2.19 "lack of progress" errors), were five times less likely to injure the gallbladder or burn non-target tissue (1 *vs*. 5 errors), and had six times fewer (84 % fewer, 1.19 *vs*. 7.38) mean errors (Fig. 11.1). These findings were confirmed in 2007 by Ahlberg et al. [62] In 2008, significantly improved performance in laparoscopic suturing after simulation-based training was observed in senior surgery residents, who had 31 % fewer errors (25.6 *vs*. 37.1) than controls, performed 34 % faster (8.8 min *vs*. 13.2 min) [63], and had 35 % fewer excess needle manipulations (18.5 *vs*. 27.3)" [63]. More recently, a 2013 assessment indicated that VR simulation-based laparoscopic skills training improved performance, and was especially effective in reducing procedural errors [64]. A systematic review of the entire body of literature on simulation-based laparoscopic surgery training to May 2014 indicated "that simulation-based training can… increase translation of laparoscopic surgery skills to the OR." Specific

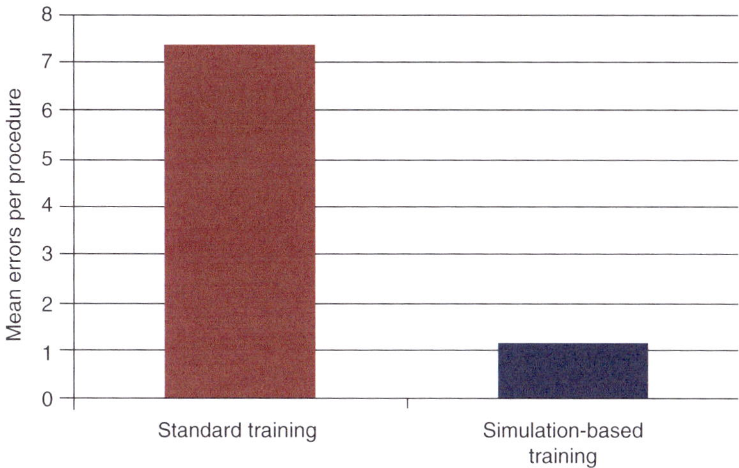

Fig. 11.1 Error reduction correlated with simulation-based training (Reprinted with permission Seymour et al. [17])

improvements included enhanced economy of movement, more accurate suturing, reduced time, and fewer errors [65].

MAS Self-Assessment

The above discussion gives a framework for thinking about self-assessment in MAS. As stated by Peyre et al., "Accurate self assessment of laparoscopic technical skill raters [66]. In another study, trainees were more self-critical and the opposite was true [39]. In other studies, surgeons' self-assessments were similar to those of raters [67, 68]. These disparities may be due to factors such as level of experience; more senior residents, for example, may be less accurate in self-assessment than junior residents [39].

Use of global rating scales can assist in self-assessment by introducing objectivity. In the Peyre et al. study, the Objective Structured Assessment of Technical Skills (OSATS) global rating scale [69] was used for self- and faculty assessments of performance of laparoscopic obstetrical and gynecology procedures [39]. The 10 technical skills in the OSATS scale were (1) preparedness, (2) respect for tissue, (3) time and motion, (4) knot tying, (5) instrument handling, (6) knowledge of instruments, (7) use of assistants, (8) anatomy, (9) knowledge of procedure, and (10) overall performance. In development can accelerate a trainee's learning growth and guide life-long development for surgeons." [39] The accuracy of self-assessment, however, is an open question. In one study, for example, surgeons' self-assessment scores after performing a laparoscopic colectomy were significantly higher than those of trained a 2011 study using OSATS, surgeons performing a laparoscopic cholecystectomy on a simulator were found to be able to accurately self-assess their technical, but not their nontechnical, skills [70].

Revalidation

In the UK and other European countries, a process of revalidation is already taking place. Revalidation is the process by which all licensed doctors have to demonstrate to the regulatory authority (General Medical Council (GMC) in the UK) that they are up to date and fit to practice. Revalidation is now a legal requirement for all doctors since its launch in the UK in December 2012, underpinned by dedicated legislation called the Medical Professional (Responsible Officers) (Amendment) Regulations 2013 [71].

The purpose of revalidation is to promote patient safety and improve the quality of patient care. It is also intended to strengthen continuing professional development and reinforce systems that identify doctors who encounter difficulties and require support. In surgery, it is intended to identify surgeons who are underperforming and surgeons are expected to provide a core set of supporting information over each revalidation cycle at appraisal. A responsible officer will assess the information from appraisal, and will then make a revalidation recommendation to the GMC, normally every five years. For full detail on the revalidation process, see the UK Revalidation Guide for Surgery [71].

Supporting Information for Surgical Revalidation

Continuing Professional Development (CPD)

The surgical Royal Colleges and specialty associations in the UK have written a CPD Summary Guide for surgery, which includes a CPD checklist, which can be used as an aid during appraisal discussions [72]. Surgeons should record their CPD in a consistent and structured way and meet some minimum requirements:

- Collect a minimum of 50 credits per year = 250 credits every 5 years
- 1 credit = 1 h of CPD
- CPD program should be set and reviewed at appraisal.

Measurement of Clinical Outcomes

The measurement of clinical outcomes of care is complex with several different methods available:

- National clinical audits specifying personal outcomes
- Outcomes derived from routinely collected data, e.g. Hospital Episode Statistics
- National clinical audits specifying the surgical team/unit's outcomes
- Local audit of outcomes
- Structured peer review of outcomes

Recertification

In the USA, the concept of time-unlimited licensure was challenged, as the public demanded some reassurance that specialists were keeping abreast of developments within their field. The American Board of Colon and Rectal Surgery (ABCRS) issued its first series of time-limited licensures in 1990, which were eventually finalized to last 10 years. The first recertification examination was administered in 1991 and by 2011, 924 participants had participated in the examination process with a 97 % pass rate [73].

The current requirements for Maintenance of Certification (MOC) [74] are as follows:

- Part I: Professional standing—Evidenced by maintaining a full and unrestricted license, providing hospital admitting and operating privileges and references from the chief of surgery and chair of credentialing.
- Part II: Life-long learning and self-assessment—Consists of Continuing Medical Education (CME) and has been revised recently so that 90 h of CME over a 3-year cycle are required, of which 60 h must be self-assessment with a post-test.
- Part III: Cognitive expertise—Passing a secure examination in the specialty at 10-year intervals. Application for the exam requires the submission of a 12-month operative log, letters of recommendation, and evidence of CME.
- Part IV: Evaluation of performance in practice—Documented through participation in outcomes database or quality-assessment programs.

MAS Accreditation

Although there is no Board certification in MAS, several professional societies have emerged to set standards in this discipline. The Society of American Gastrointestinal and Endoscopic Surgeons (SAGES, www.sages.org), founded in 1981, has become a leader in this regard. Other organizations include the Society of Laparoendoscopic Surgeons (primarily North America, www.sls.org); the Association of Laparoscopic Surgeons of Great Britain and Ireland (www.alsgbi.org), which is "the main voice for laparoscopic surgeons in the United Kingdom and Ireland"; and the World Association of Laparoscopic Surgeons (gynecology, www.wals.org.uk).

SAGES has developed the Fundamentals of Laparoscopic Surgery program (FLS, www.flsprogram.org). This "comprehensive web-based education module for laparoscopic surgery" serves as a curriculum for basic laparoscopic surgery for surgical residents, fellows, and practicing surgeons [75]. FLS includes standardized didactic information and hands-on skills training and assessment for teaching physiology, and basic MAS knowledge and technical skills. The program provides standardized MAS training, and the ability to test, measure, and document cognitive, decisionmaking, and technical skills. Because FLS is not procedure-specific, it can be used as a training adjunct in any surgical discipline. The program culminates in a test that measures cognitive knowledge, case/problem management skills and manual dexterity. Endorsed by the American College of Surgeons, FLS is accredited for CME by the ACGME. Documentation of successful completion of the FLS program is now mandatory for general surgery certification by the American Board of Surgery [76].

"We believe FLS will set the standard for laparoscopic surgery.... FLS as it provides objective evidence to residency programs that an individual resident has gained the basic knowledge and skills fundamental to the performance of laparoscopic surgery before the resident completes their [sic] program" [www.flsprogram.org].

In Europe, the European Association for Endoscopic Surgery (EAES) has developed a Laparoscopic Surgical Skills (LSS) program [77], which has the goal of provide a MAS credentialing standard [78]. The two-level program focuses on basic and advanced techniques. Within each level, participants complete a cognitive skills/knowledge pretest; simulator and scenario-based assessment of technical and nontechnical (judgment) skills, respectively; and a clinical performance assessment, which, if passed, results in LSS accreditation by the EAES.

In Japan, the Japan Society for Endoscopic Surgery (JSES) launched the Endoscopic Surgical Skill Qualification System for laparoscopic gastroenterologic surgeons [79]. Although fewer than half of the 1114 surgeons assessed by this system over a 4-year period were accredited, those who attained accreditation had a lower complication rate than those who did not. This finding led to the conclusion that the system "has impacted on the improvement and standardization of laparoscopic surgery in Japan" [79].

Conclusions

The growing demand for MAS and its steep technical learning curve, particularly for advanced procedures, emphasize the need for assessment and accreditation. When the components and types of assessment are considered in the context of MAS curriculum development, differences between cognitive and technical assessment need to be considered. Performance of MAS calls upon specific, unique skill sets, which must be practiced, and the opportunity to correct and learn from errors presented. Self-assessment is part of the MAS learning process. Lastly, the need for standardization in surgical training is being addressed by several MAS organizations, which have developed MAS curricula and accreditation mechanisms.

References

1. Suarez CA. Training, credentialing, economics and risk management in operative laparoscopy. Int Surg. 1994;79:268–72.
2. Unawane A, Kamyab A, Patel M, Flynn JC, Mittal VK. Changing paradigms in minimally invasive surgery training. Am J Surg. 2013;205:284–8.

3. Kligman M. Training considerations for laparoscopic bariatric surgery. In: National Institutes of Health, National Library of Medicine. Minimally Invasive Surgery Training: Theories, Models, Outcomes. Online book. Updated 14 May 2010. www.doc896.yuanmengying.com/laparoscopic-bariatric-surgery--P-g0lu6.pdf. Accessed 28 Apr 2015.
4. Leisner P. Surgeon says it was too late to stop amputation on wrong leg. Associated Press. 14 Sept1995.www.apnewsarchive.com/1995/Surgeon-Says-It-Was-Too-Late-to-Stop-Amputation-on-Wrong-Leg/id-a9b3238f7dbca20e0edf82bba7da0ab5. Accessed 28 Apr 2015.
5. Bristol Royal Infirmary Inquiry [Internet]. Learning from Bristol: the report of the public inquiry into children's heart surgery at the Bristol Royal Infirmary 1984–1995. Command paper: CM 5207, BRII; 2001.
6. Kohn LT, Corrigan JM, Donaldson MS, editors. To err is human: building a safer health system. Washington, DC: Institute of Medicine, National Academies Press, 2000. www.books.nap.edu/catalog.php?record_id=9728. Accessed 28 Apr 2015.
7. Finocchio LJ, Dower CM, Blick NT, et al. Strengthening consumer protection: priorities for Health Care Workforce Regulation, San Francisco; Pew Health Professions Commission, USA Oct 1998.
8. Metzger P, Gamal EM. Bile duct injuries in the era of laparoscopic cholecystectomy. Int Surg. 1995;80:328–31.
9. Deziel DJ, Millikan KW, Economou SG, Doolas A, Ko ST, Airan MC. Complications of laparoscopic cholecystectomy: a national survey of 4,292 hospitals and an analysis of 77,604 cases. Am J Surg. 1993;165:9–14.
10. Moore MJ, Bennett CL. The learning curve for laparoscopic cholecystectomy: The Southern Surgeons Club. Am J Surg. 1995;170:55–9.
11. Kumar U, Gill IS. Learning curve in human laparoscopic surgery. Curr Urol Rep. 2006;7:120–4.
12. Secin FP, Savage C, Abbou C, de La Taille A, Salomon L, Rassweiler J, et al. The learning curve for laparoscopic radical prostatectomy: an international multicenter study. J Urol. 2010;184:2291–6.
13. Larsen CR, Soerensen JL, Grantcharov TP, Dalsgaard T, Schouenborg L, Ottosen C, Schroeder TV, Ottesen BS. Effect of virtual reality training on laparoscopic surgery: randomised controlled trial. BMJ 2009;338:b1802. www.bmj.com/content/338/bmj.b1802.pdf%2Bhtml. Accessed 28 Apr 2015.
14. Hamad GG, Curet M. Minimally invasive surgery. Am J Surg. 2010,199:263–5.
15. Fried GM, Feldman LS, Vassiliou MC, Fraser SA, Stanbridge D, Ghitulescu G, et al. Proving the value of simulation in laparoscopic surgery. Ann Surg. 2004;240:518–25; discussion 525–8.
16. Stefanidis D, Sevdalis N, Paige J, Zevin B, Aggarwal R, Grantcharov T, Jones DB. Simulation in surgery: what's needed next? Ann Surg. 2015;261:846–53.
17. Seymour NE, Gallagher AG, Roman SA, O'Brien MK, Bansal VK, Andersen DK, et al. Virtual reality training improves OR performance: results of a randomized, double-blinded study. Ann Surg. 2002;236:458–63; discussion 463–4.
18. Cannon WD, Garrett Jr WE, Hunter RE, Sweeney HJ, Eckhoff DG, Nicandri GT, et al. Improving residency training in arthroscopic knee surgery with use of a virtual-reality simulator. A randomized blinded study. J Bone Joint Surg Am. 2014;96:1798–806.
19. Gomez PP, Willis RE, Van Sickle K. Evaluation of two flexible colonoscopy simulators and transfer of skills into clinical practice. J Surg Educ. 2015;72:220–7.
20. Zerey M, Harrell AG, Kercher KW, Heniford BT. Minimally invasive surgery training overview. In National Institutes of Health, National Library of Medicine. Minimally Invasive Surgery Training: Theories, Models, Outcomes. Updated 14 May 2010.
21. Ghaderi I, Auvergne L, Park YS, Farrell TM. Quantitative and qualitative analysis of performance during advanced laparoscopic fellowship: a curriculum based on structured assessment and feedback. Am J Surg. 2015;209:71–8.
22. Gallagher AG, Ritter EM, Champion H, Higgins G, Fried MP, Moses G, et al. Virtual reality simulation for the operating room: proficiency-based training as a paradigm shift in surgical skills training. Ann Surg. 2005;242:364–72.

23. Rukovets O. Simulation-based mastery learning more effective than clinical experience for lumbar puncture. Neurol Today. 2012:7–8.
24. Jordan J, Gallagher A, McGuigan J, McClure N. Virtual reality training leads to faster adaptation to the novel psychomotor restrictions encountered by laparoscopic surgeons. Surg Endosc. 2001;15:1080–4.
25. Gallagher H, Allan J, Tolley D. Spatial awareness in urologists: are they different? BJU Int. 2001;88:666–70.
26. Madan A, Frantzides C. Substituting virtual reality trainers for inanimate box trainers does not decrease laparoscopic skills acquisition. J Soc Laparoendosc Surg. 2007;11:87–9.
27. Pearson A, Gallagher A, Rosser J, Satava R. Evaluation of structured and quantitative training methods for teaching intracorporeal knot tying. Surg Endosc. 2002;16:130–7.
28. McLaughlin S, Fitch MT, Goyal DG, Hayden E, Yang Kauh C, Laack TA, et al. Simulation in graduate medical education 2008: a review for emergency medicine. Acad Emerg Med. 2008;15:1117–29.
29. Issenberg SB, McGaghie WC. Clinical skills training–practice makes perfect. Med Educ. 2002;36:210.
30. Ericsson KA. Deliberate practice and the acquisition and maintenance of expert performance in medicine and related domains. Acad Med. 2004;79(Suppl):S70–81.
31. Subhas G, Mittal VK. Minimally invasive training during surgical residency. Am Surg. 2011;77:902–6.
32. Kirkpatrick DL. Evaluation of training. In: Craig RL, editor. Training and development handbook: a guide to human resource development. New York: McGraw Hill; 1976.
33. Bandura A. Guide for constructing self-efficacy scales. In: Pajares F, Urdan T, editors. Adolescence and Education, Volume V: Self-efficacy beliefs of adolescents. Greenwich: Information Age Publishing; 2006. http://www.uky.edu/~eushe2/Bandura/BanduraGuide2006.pdf. Accessed 28 Apr 2015.
34. Chen G, Gully SM, Eden D. Validation of a new general self-efficacy scale. Organ Res Meth. 2001;4(1):62–83.
35. Baldwin TT, Ford J. Transfer of training: a review and directions for future research. Personnel Psychol. 1988;41:63–105.
36. Wass V, Van der Vleuten C, Shatzer J, Jones R. Assessment of clinical competence. Lancet. 2001;357:95–949. http://acmd615.pbworks.com/f/Wass.pdf. Accessed 27 Feb 2013.
37. Handfield-Jones RS, Mann KV, Challis ME, Hobma SO, Klass DJ. McManus IC, Paget NS, Parboosingh IJ, Wade WB, Wilkinson TJ. Linking assessment to learning: a new route to quality assurance in medical practice. Med Educ. 2002;36:949–58. www.ucl.ac.uk/medical-education/reprints/2002MedEd--Linking_assessmentToLearning.pdf. Accessed 28 Apr 2015.
38. Mitra NK, Barua A. Effect of online formative assessment on summative performance in integrated musculoskeletal system module. BMC Med Educ. 2015;15:29–35. http://www.ncbi.nlm.nih.gov/pmc/articles/PMC4351696/pdf/12909_2015_Article_318.pdf. Accessed 28 Apr 2015.
39. Peyre SE, MacDonald H, Al-Marayati L, Templeman C, Muderspach LI. Resident self-assessment versus faculty assessment of laparoscopic technical skills using a global rating scale. Int J Med Educ. 2010;1:37–41.
40. Payandeh S, Lomax AJ, Dill J, Mackenzie CL, Cao CGL. On defining metrics for assessing laparoscopic surgical skills in a virtual training environment. MMVR. 2002. http://cecs.wright.edu/sites/default/files/erel/2002_OnDefiningMetrics.pdf. Accessed 28 Apr 2015.
41. Payandeh S, Lomax A. A Knotting theory and knotting mechanisms. Proceedings of ASME 25th Biennial Mechanisms Conference. Atlanta, Georgia. USA 1998.
42. Cao CGL, MacKenzie CL, Payandeh S. Task and motion analysis in endoscopic surgery. Proceedings of ASME dynamic systems, 5th annual symposium on haptic interface for virtual environment and teleoperation. Atlanta, Georgia. USA 1996.

43. Stanisic Z, Jackson E, Payandeh S. Virtual fixtures as an aid for teleoperation. Proceedings of 9th Canadian Aeronautic and Space Institute Conference. Canada 1996.
44. Royal Australasian College of Surgeons, The College of Surgeons of Australia and New Zealand. Surgical competence and performance: a guide to the assessment and development of surgeons, 2nd ed. 2011. https://www.surgeons.org/media/18955288/surgical_competence_and_performance_guide__2011_.pdf. Accessed 28 Apr 2015.
45. Liang H, Shi M. Quality assessment in virtual surgical training. In: Applied informatics and communication. International Conference, ICAIC 2011, Xi'an, August 20–21, 2011, Proceedings Part I. p. 330–7.
46. Cundy TP, Thangaraj E, Rafii-Tari H, Payne CJ, Azzie G, Sodergren MH, et al. Force-sensing enhanced simulation environment (ForSense) for laparoscopic surgery training and assessment. Surgery. 2015;157(4):723–31.
47. Raghu Prasad MS, Manivannan M, Chandramohan SM. Effects of laparoscopic instrument and finger on force perception: a first step towards laparoscopic force-skills training. Surg Endosc. 2015;29(7):1927–43.
48. Singapogu RB, Smith DC, Long LO, Burg TC, Pagano CC, Burg KJ. Objective differentiation of force-based laparoscopic skills using a novel haptic simulator. J Surg Educ. 2012;69:766–73.
49. Champion HR, Meglan DA, Shair EK. Minimizing surgical error by incorporating objective assessment into surgical education. J Am Coll Surg. 2008;207:284–91.
50. Kirsch G. Learning from our medical mistakes. Canadian College of Health Service Executives; 2005.
51. Kao LS. Error analysis in minimally invasive surgery training. In: National Institutes of Health, National Library of Medicine. Minimally invasive surgery training: theories, models, outcomes. Updated 14 May 2010.
52. Way LW, Stewart L, Gantert W, Liu K, Lee CM, Whang K, et al. Causes and prevention of laparoscopic bile duct injuries: analysis of 252 cases from a human factors and cognitive psychology perspective. Ann Surg. 2003;237:460–9.
53. Flum DR, Cheadle A, Prela C, Dellinger EP, Chan L. Bile duct injury during cholecystectomy and survival in medicare beneficiaries. JAMA. 2003;290:2168–73.
54. Regenbogen SE, Greenberg CC, Studdert DM, et al. Patterns of technical error among surgical malpractice claims: an analysis of strategies to prevent injury to surgical patients. Ann Surg. 2007;246:705–11.
55. Healey MA, Shackford SR, Osler TM, et al. Complications in surgical patients. Arch Surg. 2002;137:611–8.
56. Bates DW, O'Neill AC, Peterson LA, et al. Evaluation of screening criteria for adverse events in medical patients. Med Care. 1995;33:452–62.
57. Wilson RM, Runciman WB, Gibberd RW, et al. The quality in Australian health care study. Med J Aust. 1995;163:459–71.
58. Brennan TA, Leape LL, Laird NM, et al. Incidence of adverse events and negligence in hospitalized patients: results of the harvard medical practice study I. N Engl J Med. 1991;324:370–6.
59. Andrews LB, Stocking C, Krizek T, et al. An alternative strategy for studying adverse events in medical care. Lancet. 1997;349:309–13.
60. McGuire HH, Horsley III JS, Salter DR, Sobel M. Measuring and managing quality of surgery: statistical vs. incidental approaches. Arch Surg. 1992;127:733–7.
61. Thomas EJ, Studdert DM, Burstin HR, et al. Incidence and types of adverse events and negligent car in Utah and Colorado. Med Care. 2000;38:261–71.
62. Ahlberg G, Enochsson L, Gallagher AG, et al. Proficiency-based virtual reality training significantly reduces the error rate for residents during their first 10 laparoscopic cholecystectomies. Am J Surg. 2007;193:797–804.
63. Van Sickle KR, Ritter EM, Baghai M, Goldenberg AE, Huang IP, Gallagher AG, Smith CD. Prospective, randomized, double-blind trial of curriculum-based training for intracorporeal suturing and knot tying. J Am Coll Surg. 2008;207:560–8.

64. Gallagher AG, Seymour NE, Jordan-Black JA, Bunting BP, McGlade K, Satava RM. Prospective, randomized assessment of transfer of training (ToT) and transfer effectiveness ratio (TER) of virtual reality simulation training for laparoscopic skill acquisition. Ann Surg. 2013;257(6):1025–31.
65. Vanderbilt AA, Grover AC, Pastis NJ, Feldman M, Granados DD, Murithi LK, Mainous 3rd AG. Randomized controlled trials: a systematic review of laparoscopic surgery and simulation-based training. Glob J Health Sci. 2014;7:310–27.
66. Sidhu RS, Vikis E, Cheifetz R, Phang T. Self-assessment during a 2-day laparoscopic colectomy course: can surgeons judge how well they are learning new skills? Am J Surg. 2006;191:677–81.
67. Sarker SK, Chang A, Vincent C. Technical and technological skills assessment in laparoscopic surgery. J Soc Laparoend Surg. 2006;10:284–92.
68. Sarker SK, Hutchinson R, Chang A, Vincent C, Darzi AW. Self-appraisal hierarchical task analysis of laparoscopic surgery performed by expert surgeons. Surg Endosc. 2006;20: 636–40.
69. Martin JA, Regehr G, Reznick R, MacRae H, Murnaghan J, Hutchinson C, et al. Objective structured assessment of technical skills (OSATS) for surgical residents. Br J Surg. 1997;84:273–8.
70. Arora S, Miskovic D, Hull L, Moorthy K, Aggarwal R, Johannsson H, Gautama S, Kneebone R, Sevdalis N. Self vs expert assessment of technical and non-technical skills in high fidelity simulation. Am J Surg. 2011;202:500–6.
71. General Medical Council-UK 2013. http://www.gmcuk.org/doctors/revalidation/revalidation_gmp_framework.asp.
72. Revalidation Guide for Surgery. Federation of Surgical Specialty Associations | The Royal College of Surgeons of Edinburgh The Royal College of Surgeons UK. 2014. http://www.rcseng.ac.uk/surgeons/surgicalstandards/docs/revalidation-guide-for-surgery.
73. Schoetz DJ. The American Board of colon and rectal surgery: past, present, and future. Clin Colon Rectal Surg. 2012;25(3):166–70. doi:10.1055/s-0032-1322554.
74. Luchtefeld M, Kerwel TG. Continuing medical education, maintenance of certification, and physician reentry. Clin Colon Rectal Surg. 2012;25(3):171–6. doi:10.1055/s-0032-1322546.
75. Fundamentals of Laparoscopic Surgery website. 2013. http://www.flsprogram.org. Accessed 28 Apr 2015.
76. Training requirements for general surgery certification. www.absurgery.org/default.jsp?certgsqe_training. Accessed 28 Apr 2015.
77. Buzink S, Soltes M, Radonak J, Fingerhut A, Hanna G, Jakimowicz J. Laparoscopic surgical skills programme: preliminary evaluation of grade I level 1 courses by trainees. Wideochir Inne Tech Malo Inwazyjne. 2012;7(3):188–192. http://www.ncbi.nlm.nih.gov/pmc/articles/PMC3516988/#CIT0003. Accessed 28 Apr 2015.
78. Laparoscopic Surgical Skills Foundation. 2011. http://www.lss-surgical.eu. Accessed 28 Apr 2015.
79. Mori T, Kimura T, Kitajima M. Skill accreditation system for laparoscopic gastroenterologic surgeons in Japan. Minim Invasive Ther Allied Technol. 2010;19(1):18–23.

Chapter 12
Training the Trainer in Laparoscopic Surgery

Mark Coleman and Nader Francis

Introduction

Surgery used to be a cognitive apprenticeship that comprised the gradual acquisition of knowledge, skills and behaviours under the supervision of an expert trainer. Never before has the effectiveness of surgery and the safety been more closely scrutinized by the public [1, 2]. It is no longer acceptable for trainee surgeons to learn unsupervised; confirmation of competence is a vital pre-requisite to independent performance.

Enhancing the quality of surgical training to achieve competency has received much more attention recently, particularly within Minimal Access Surgery (MAS), due to its known prolonged long proficiency-gain curve and shortening of training time in this technically challenging field [3–6].

MAS, however, affords the best opportunity for both the direct and retrospective observation of surgical performance compared to traditional open surgery. It also provides an accurate means to objectively scrutinize the contribution of a trainer to the performance of a surgical procedure. Optimum surgical performance requires a combination of knowledge, technical skills and behaviour [7]. For index procedures and parts of procedures, within the sub-specialty of MAS, the performance of trainees can be observed by using a structured pre-determined assessment format to assess the acquisition of skills [8]. Beyond the process of learning the technical skills themselves, are the less tangible elements of the enhancement of knowledge and behaviours essential to the development of a surgeon. Surgical training has

M. Coleman
Consultant Colorectal Surgeon, Derriford Hospital, Plymouth, UK

N. Francis, MB ChB, PLAB, FRCS, PhD (✉)
Colorectal Surgery, Yeovil District Hospital NHS Foundation Trust,
Higher Kingston Yeovil, Somerset BA21 4AT, UK
e-mail: Nader.francis@ydh.nhs.uk

N. Francis et al. (eds.), *Training in Minimal Access Surgery*,
DOI 10.1007/978-1-4471-6494-4_12

changed from a craft apprenticeship, where skills were acquired gradually by observation and practice, to a more structured competency-based approach [9–11].

This chapter explores the process of becoming a trainer in MAS in terms of understanding the technical and non-technical skills that underpin optimum teaching, the best structure for training and the most efficient way to improve teaching in MAS.

What Makes "a Great Trainer"?

Not all surgeons make good trainers. Some great surgeons are poor performers when it comes to the transference of their own knowledge, skills and behaviour to junior colleagues.

In recent years, there has been an increased awareness and better understanding of the importance of communication, teamwork and the effect of so-called non-technical skills on clinical outcome, as opposed to simply learning the practical skills [12–14]. For an adult to learn a practical skill effectively, the trainer needs to be aware of the trainee's needs. This involves the amount of new information that is imparted to ensure that the trainee maintains motivation, continues to progress and does not suffer from cognitive overload, whilst remaining mindful that the training episode does not affect patient safety.

Nevertheless, within MAS a high level of technical skill is required for optimum surgical performance. Often in MAS, a long proficiency-gain curve prohibits a self-taught approach, with evidence that supervised teaching promotes a better patient outcome [15]. It is well known that, in general, there is a lack of uniformity in operative approach amongst surgeons and surgical faculty. Although there are essential steps in the performance of MAS, some surgeons execute certain tasks in different ways, often due to being self-taught. Little is known about whether there is a consensus about the "right" way to structure the training of MAS. The provision of high quality teaching is imperative to maximise the chance of trainees acquiring proficiency in new skills and procedures, and different trainers have been shown to impact on trainees' performance, even in basic skills.

With prior experience in teaching and education in MAS, we can summarise that the basic general characteristics of a good trainer can include, competency in the task, enthusiasm, confidence, clear and well-organized presentation of instructional material, skill in interaction with students/residents individually or in group settings. It is also important to involve the trainee in the teaching process, have a humanistic or empathic orientation, a good knowledge of the subject and most importantly, be learner-focused, inspiring and a role model.

The Training the Trainer Curriculum

Teaching methods have been evaluated within some specialties of medicine· but none of these have been designed for use with peers or senior trainee surgery [16]. In endoscopy, however, a highly regarded Training the Colonoscopy

Trainers (TCT) was developed by the UK National Joint Advisory Group for Gastrointestinal Endoscopy (JAG) to provide a training framework for teaching endoscopy [17] (Chap. 5). In MAS, an adapted model was developed based on the TCT and modified to be applied and validated in laparoscopic colorectal surgery for over 70 national trainers within the Lapco National Training programme in England [18].

This course was set out to explain the means whereby a more structured, reflective and cognitive approach to training is likely to improve the training process. Although the course is bespoke to laparoscopic colorectal surgery, it is highly applicable to other specialties in MAS. The basis for Lapco TT in laparoscopic surgery is to provide a framework of training in order to maximise every opportunity from before, during and after training occurs. This starts with pre-operative preparation, which is termed 'Set', the process that occurs during the MAS procedure itself termed 'Dialogue', and the period after the procedure termed 'Closure'. The full details of this framework are already covered in Chap. 5, but the application of each section of the framework in laparoscopic training will be examined here.

Pre-operative Preparation: The 'Set'

Physical Set

The physical set in laparoscopy is defined here as the layout of the Operating Room (OR) and the function of all the manpower and equipment therein. Although no two operating rooms are alike, the position and function of all its human and non-human resources are vital to the safe, effective and efficient performance of MAS. Moreover, MAS is arguably more dependent on such factors than open surgery. An effective trainer needs to be a highly skilled to make the OR environment more conducive to training. In MAS, trainees are often more drawn into on the technical details of the procedure itself, without checking the optimum physical set and ergonomics and how these factors can be crucial on their performance and learning.

The factors that are keys to the physical set are:

- Laparoscopic stack placement
- Appropriate settings for gas insufflation, energy devices and camera/light controls and all ergonomics of laparoscopic instruments
- Patient and table positioning
- Personnel placement in the OR relative to the patient, each other and the equipment

By leading the physical set the trainer not only demonstrates to and involves the trainee in optimal OR setup, but also makes sure the procedure runs smoothly and acts as a good role model for the whole team prior to the start of the procedure. Modern ORs often have integrated equipment that can facilitate the physical set. The position of the trainer in the OR is also worthy of consideration. Depending on the level, confidence and expectations of the trainer and trainee will determine whether the trainer is scrubbed or un-scrubbed in the OR.

Alignment of Agendas

This is the process whereby trainer and trainee integrate a common understanding for a planned training episode. The training episode might include a placement or prolonged period, an operating list, or an individual case. Both trainer and trainee need to have a constructive dialogue about the trainee's prior experience, capabilities, confidence and expectations. This discussion can be used to form an agreement as to how the subsequent training episode will proceed. It should include consideration by the trainer and trainee as to what the trainee can reasonably expect to be able to do, taking into account prior experience. The objective of alignment of agendas is to obtain a clear common understanding and the benefit is that both avoid disappointment when undisclosed expectations are not achieved.

Alignment of agendas includes the following:

- Review trainee's prior experience
- Review trainee's most recent learning objective
- Agree on a training plan for the placement, operating list or individual case
- Ground rules

Prior to the start of a training episode it is vital that the trainer and trainee have a clear understanding of the language of training. This is not only necessary for patient safety, but vital so that there is unequivocal communication between the trainee and trainer. Simple commands such as 'stop' need prior discussion to avoid disappointment in the trainee, who might misunderstand that the training opportunity is over. In MAS, directions from the trainer to the trainee with regards to MAS instrument path and directions need prior explanation and agreement to avoid confusion. Examples include discussion of the word 'Stop' (mentioned above) and whether directional commands such as up, down, left and right refer to hand movements or screen movements. In MAS there is potential for confusion due to the fulcrum effect of the instruments and to avoid confusion instructions should be referred to the monitor view, rather than focusing on hand movements. The setting of ground rules can also include the camera assistant.

It is crucial in training to adhere to the process of the preparation or "SET" prior to commencing the actual coaching. Although this process can take a long time at the initial phase between trainers and their new trainees, it can take only a few minutes especially between trainers and trainees who are familiar with each other. Alignment of agendas should take place before each case to agree on clear mutual objectives, no matter how long the trainer and trainee have been working together.

The Procedure: The 'Dialogue"

The 'dialogue' is the process of clinical coaching in the OR that occurs during a procedure. It should only occur after all aspects of the 'set' are complete. The dialogue involves whether the trainer is scrubbed or not, where the trainer is positioned and whether the trainer plays a physical role in the procedure or not. Clear, concise, common language is required to avoid confusion.

Effective clinical coaching in advanced laparoscopic surgery requires 3 important key teaching skills:

1. Conscious competence as a trainer
2. Performance Enhancing Instruction
3. A structured approach to avoid taking over

Conscious Competence (Fig. 12.1)

Competence is defined as performing the task safely and within a reasonable timeframe [19]. The concept of conscious competence has been noted in medical education where learners moving from conscious competence, where they can perform a technique but have to think about it, to unconscious competence where they have acquired mastery of the technique and no longer have to think about it [20]. However, it is worth saying here that a trainee without adequate insight might have 'Unconscious Incompetence'; a lack of awareness that they are unable to perform a procedure satisfactorily. That insight should be provided by the trainer. Through a process of training by the acquisition and application of skills and knowledge, the trainee becomes 'Consciously Competent'; they are aware that they can perform the procedure and each of the key steps therein. As they progress further they can develop the skill to perform the procedure, which is to say, they can perform the procedure without deconstruction – 'Unconscious Competence'. All competent

Unconscious Incompetence **UI** Junior trainee	**Conscious Incompetence** **CI** More experienced trainee or Fellow in difficult tasks
Unconscious Competence **UC** Experienced surgeon Perform tasks automatically without thinking	**Conscious Competence** **CC** Consciously able to deconstruct the procedure to trainee The trainer needs to be in this box to be a good trainer

Fig. 12.1 Stages of learning

surgeons will have a limit to their competency and will be conscious of that limit; the boundary where they go from competence to incompetence. In most cases they have the insight and situational awareness to know the limit and seek help. A good example would be a situation that requires a different surgical expertise.

Conscious Competence as a Trainer

The same model of conscious competence can be applied to the ability of a trainer. Most trainers are accomplished surgical experts who can perform MAS procedures without thought; they are 'Unconsciously Competent' for most cases they perform. This is not a useful realm to be in as a trainer. A good trainer is one who can deconstruct each task and train by explanation and demonstration, in other words be a 'Consciously Competent Trainer'. The more a trainer remains consciously competent, the greater the chances trainees have to acquire skills. Of course, as a trainee progresses to conscious competence themselves, the trainer, though still present, no longer needs to explain and deconstruct. Equally if a trainee cannot perform a part of a procedure, the trainer may not be able to proceed with the training episode without taking over temporarily – this can be defined as conscious incompetence as a trainer. Hopefully by deconstruction and/or taking over, conscious competence as a trainer can be restored such that control can be handed back to the trainee to allow the training to proceed. We explore taking over in the OR in the next section.

Performance Enhancing Instruction

This section explores examples of the effects of different levels of verbal instruction from a trainer to a trainee during a surgical procedure. During the process of training, different types of verbal instruction are used. It is necessary for trainers to have a good understanding of the effects of differing instruction on the trainee's ability. This can be divided into 5 levels (Fig. 12.2). Level 1 is where no comment or instruction is provided by the trainer to the trainee. Although this might be completely appropriate where a trainee is competent to proceed, level 1 instruction will be unlikely to obtain any learning benefit. Level 2 is negative criticism (e.g. 'that's rubbish!', or 'that's not how I do it'). Other than in a light-hearted context, level 2 is likely to be detrimental to both morale and performance and can impact negatively on the trainee's confidence. Although, it is understandable that in certain occasions, criticism may be required, this needs to be carried out in a constructive way, rather than in a patronizing and insulting manner. Level 3 is positive but non-specific (e.g. 'that's great, well done!', or 'you're the best!'). This level might help morale, but is also unlikely to result in an improvement, as it lacks clarity on what exactly they have achieved well. Level 4 is instruction that is directive but not specific or focused, which entails providing some instructions but perhaps vague and non-specific (e.g. 'up a bit, down a bit, left, right'). Finally, level 5 is directive, specific and focused. Equally important in level 5 is to ask questions of the trainee: 'what do you need to know?', or 'are you

Level	Faculty comments
Level 1	No Comment
Level 2	Critic without explanation, negative non-specific (That was rubbish!)
Level 3	No Directions–positive, non specific (Well done!)
Level 4	Some directions, but not specific (bit more left or right)
Level 5	Directive, specific and focused

Fig. 12.2 Levels of instructions during coaching

happy with my instructions?' By using level 5 instruction, the coaching would be trainee-focused and the performance of the trainee is more likely to be optimal.

Strategy to Avoid Taking Over

One of the main challenges in surgical training is to avoid a situation where the trainer takes over the procedure from the trainee, thereby depriving the latter of a valuable training opportunity. This section explores the moment where the performance of an operation is interrupted by the trainer whose temptation is to take over. The aim of this session is to promote the adoption of a framework whereby this might be avoided.

Lack of progress during surgical training usually occurs when a trainee cannot proceed safely. This might be identified by either the trainer or trainee. The trainee might be aware of the reasons for inability to proceed or the trainer might halt the procedure. In MAS this is most often due to anatomical uncertainty, an inadequate view or a lack of ability to interpret the anatomy from the screen. In many instances the trainer will take over, often for the remainder of the procedure, thus losing a valuable training opportunity for the trainee. If the reason for failure to progress can be identified and resolved without taking over, the training episode can proceed and will benefit the trainee.

The first step (see Fig. 12.3) is to stop the procedure. Stopping or rather pausing the procedure should be agreed on during the "SET" phase as an opportunity to explain the causes of the lack of progress. Trainees need to understand that, when the trainer is asking them to stop it is not offending them, but rather to discuss progress or the lack of it. The second step is to ask the trainee to identify the reason that this part of the procedure is not going as planned. The third step is for the trainer to explain the reason for the problem if the trainee failed to identify the reason(s) and develop a matched

6 POINT INSTRUCTION	CONVERSATION WITH THE TRAINEE
1. STOP	Give the command
2. IDENTIFY	Ask the trainee to tell you what they are doing?
3. EXPLAIN	What do you think the reason is for stopping? The trainee needs to think what is going on
4. INSTRUCT	Tell them what you want them to do
5. CHECK	Ask them to tell you what they are going to do now?
6. JUDGE	Is it OK for the trainee to proceed? Continue with the procedure

Fig. 12.3 6 point process to avoid taking over in theatre

understanding. The fourth is for the trainer to instruct the trainee how to proceed in such a way as to rectify the problem. The fifth is for the trainee to explain how they plan to proceed and for the trainer check that their explanation in steps three and four has been understood. Finally in step 6 the trainee recommences the procedure and the trainer judges the trainee's capability to proceed. If progress from that point remains hesitant, it might be necessary to repeat the six-point plan more than once as required.

By using this six-point plan accompanied by good preparation in the 'Set', the trainer is less likely to take over and the trainee more likely to benefit for the training episode

Post-operative: The 'Closure' or Feedback

Feedback is a vital part of training [21]. The main priorities are to reflect on the procedure just completed and develop learning objectives that are likely to result in improvements in future performance.

For psycho-motor skills acquisition, feedback is the foundation of effective training and is considered one of the most important variables, aside from practice [21].

There are two types of feedback [22]:

- Concurrent feedback: which is referred to the feedback received during the performance and is covered in the previous section (performance enhancing instructions).
- Terminal feedback, which is referred to the feedback provided after the completion of the task. The potential use of terminal feedback as a learning tool in simulation-based surgical training is significant and results in better learning

when compared to concurrent feedback. The downfall of terminal feedback in clinical settings is that errors cannot be allowed to progress due to patient safety.

Feedback Model in LAPCO TT

There are a number of ways to provide feedback, which have been discussed in Chap. 5. However, we will examine here the model, which was adopted for the LAPCO TT programme. Feedback can take place after a single procedure, operating list or training placement. Often service pressures result in feedback being overlooked, but it is a vital opportunity to summarize and crystallize a training episode in such a way that is likely to result in performance improvement.

The means whereby this can be achieved is to start by shared reflection between the trainer and trainee to gain an understanding of how the procedure went. Usually this takes the form of a question from trainer to trainee: "how do you think that went?'. This allows the trainee to reflect on their performance and allows the trainer to see whether the trainee's perspective matches their own. This is often followed by an exploration of the trainer's perspective: 'yes, I agree, that went well'. Then, the trainer asks the trainee to reflect on the areas of difficulty and allow them to analyse and identify the reasons, come up with learning objectives and take-home messages. There should be only one or two main points that they need to focus on for the next cases.

For feedback to be effective there are several considerations to take into account:

- The physical environment where feedback takes place. Ideally this should be quiet and confidential, so the trainer and trainee can engage in a frank discussion without being overheard.
- The feedback session should be a two-way process, whereby both the trainer and trainee discuss the training episode openly. The session should start with a question from the trainer: for example, 'how do think that went?' This allows the trainer and trainee to align agendas and gain a common understanding.
- Video feedback may be used to analyze the performance. A critical aspect in the video feedback involves directing the attention of the trainee to specific aspects of the performance that require modification or correction to improve focus.
- Feedback should have the objective of delivering a simple understandable message or learning objective for the trainee to improve subsequent performance.

Other Training Issues in MAS

Dual Task Interference

All humans have a variable but limited capacity to perform manual tasks [23]. The more familiar the task and the more practiced the individual, the more the ability to maintain performance in the presence of additional sensory stimuli. It is expected, therefore, that novices to MAS will be more susceptible to reduced performance in the presence of interference. The presence of interference that is not in itself required in the operating room is likely to reduce the performance of the trainee. Examples of interference are most often auditory, including music, conversation, radio pagers and telephones, or visual including movement of people or objects in the field of vision of the trainee, or even in front of the laparoscopic television monitor. The trainer will most often have a higher level of authority and situational awareness than the trainee and a good trainer will effectively control the operating room to reduce interference with the trainee.

Assessment and Accreditation

This is covered separately in Chap. 11, but in this chapter, will focus on the assessment tools that were used in LAPCO programme, including the formative and summative tools.

Formative Assessment

Within LAPCO, a bespoke assessment tool was created to monitor progression and proficiency gain in laparoscopic colorectal surgery – the Global Assessment Scale (GAS) [24]. This is a formative tool, which divides laparoscopic colorectal operations into twelve steps, which are rated by both the trainee and the trainer immediately after the case, using an objective scoring scale. The scale differs from many assessment tools in that it uses statements describing the degree of independence with which the step was performed by the trainee, rather than more subjective judgmental descriptors of how well it was performed such as "good" or "poor performance." The form was used after every training case to structure feedback, and it allows areas of weakness and strength to be identified and a trainee's progress to be tracked. The GAS tool has since been adopted by surgical trainees in the UK outside the LAPCO programme, in particular those undertaking fellowship and residency training in laparoscopic colorectal surgery [25].

Summative Assessment

A ***summative*** assessment tool was developed for sign-off of surgeons from the LAPCO program. Trainees were required to submit two DVDs showing a right and a left sided colon resection. The Laparoscopic Competency Assessment Tool (L-CAT) was designed to provide a framework of objective criteria to facilitate objective evaluation of the DVD by blinded expert assessors [26]. Construct validity at the specialist level has been demonstrated, with the tool capable of differentiating between experts and trainees, and also between those trainees who the experts felt should pass the assessment versus those who did not pass.

Human Factors and Training

Human factors is discussed in details in a separate chapter (Chap. 14). However, within the context of training the trainer 'Human factors' is the process of learning where we try to understand and improve the roles of individuals and teams involved in healthcare with the objective of trying to reduce the incidence of harmful incidents. The contributions of surgical trainers as individuals and their teams they work in are complex and multi-factorial. All individuals have their own innate personalities, developed at an early age. These personalities have a key impact on the way a team works. Day to day behaviour might be different from how individuals like to behave naturally and is influenced by a number of factors. Selecting and maintaining appropriate behaviours are essential to the effective discharge of individual and collective professional responsibilities. Key to the function of a team is effective leadership in MAS and equally effective followership.

The human factors that influence the functional effectiveness of a team are as follows [14]:

- **Communication** – managing professional to professional communication in a safety-critical environment
- **Situation Awareness** – the often flawed process of understanding what is 'going on'
- **Risk Management** – how we can discharge our responsibility to reduce risk and harm
- **Personality** and its impact on performance and team working
- **Human Factors Feedback** – regulating those behaviours as an everyday process
- **Managing overload and using the tools** – staying in control in stressful situations or extremely risky environments and making briefings, debriefings, handovers and checklists work effectively
- **Leading, Following and Motivating** – our professional responsibilities to everyone else in the team

Summary

Training in MAS presents unique challenges compared to training in open surgery: loss of tactile sense, lack of 3D visuo-spatial awareness, greater reliance on the non-dominant hand and reduced ability for the trainer to facilitate the procedure by traction and counter-traction. Yet there are also distinct advantages: magnified and high definition views of the operative field, the potential to train without being scrubbed and the ability to video record procedures easily for subsequent reflection and independent review. As with all surgical training, the key elements should not be forgotten: conscious competence as a surgeon and a trainer, empathy, patience, communication skills, leadership, organisation, situational awareness and emotional intelligence. Structured, validated and reliable forms of formative and summative assessment enable performance enhancing feedback and allow high fidelity observation of the proficiency-gain curve for individual trainees and groups of trainees.

The lessons learnt from LAPCO, a performance-managed transformational national training programme for laparoscopic colorectal surgery, can be applied in any healthcare system or region and can be reproduced in all specialties of MAS.

References

1. Kligman M. Training considerations for laparoscopic bariatric surgery. In: National Institutes of Health, National Library of Medicine. Minimally Invasive Surgery Training: Theories, Models, Outcomes. Online book. http://mastri.umm.edu/NIH-Book/training_bariatric.html. Accessed May 2013.
2. Bristol Royal Infirmary Inquiry [Internet]. Learning from Bristol: The report of the public inquiry into children's heart surgery at the Bristol Royal Infirmary 1984–1995. Command paper: CM 5207, BRII; 2001. http://www.bristol-inquiry.org.uk/final_report/the_report.pdf. Accessed 5 Mar 2013.
3. Deziel DJ, Millikan KW, Economou SG, Doolas A, Ko ST, Airan MC. Complications of laparoscopic cholecystectomy: a national survey of 4,292 hospitals and an analysis of 77,604 cases. Am J Surg. 1993;165:9–14.
4. Moore MJ, Bennett CL. The learning curve for laparoscopic cholecystectomy: The Southern Surgeons Club. Am J Surg. 1995;170:55–9.
5. Kumar U, Gill IS. Learning curve in human laparoscopic surgery. Curr Urol Rep. 2006;7:120–4.
6. Secin FP, Savage C, Abbou C, de La Taille A, Salomon L, Rassweiler J, Hruza M, Rozet F, Cathelineau X, Janetschek J, Nassar F, Turk I, Vanni AJ, Gill IS, Koenig P, Kaouk JH, Pineiro LM, Pansadoro V, Emiliozzi P, Bjartell A, Jiborn T, Eden C, Richards AJ, Van Velthoven R, Stolzenburg J-U, Rabenalt R, Su L-M, Pavlovich CP, Levinson AW, Touijer KA, Vickers A, Guillonneau B. The learning curve for laparoscopic radical prostatectomy: an international multicenter study. J Urol. 2010;184:2291–6.
7. Gowande AA. Creating the educated surgeon in the 21st century. Am J Surg. 2001;181:551–6.
8. van Sickle KR, Gallagher AG, Smith CD. The effect of escalating feedback on the acquisition of psychomotor skills for laparoscopy. Surg Endosc. 2007;21:220–4.
9. American Board of Surgery, available at http://www.absurgery.org/default.jsp?certgsqe_resassess. Last accessed 14 July 2014.
10. Larson JL, Williams RG, Ketchum J, Boehler ML, Dunnington GL. Feasibility, reliability and validity of an operative performance rating system for evaluating surgery residents. Surgery. 2005;138(4):640–7.
11. Intercollegiate Surgical Curriculum Project, available at: https://www.iscp.ac.uk. Last accessed 14 July 2014.
12. Siu J, Maran N, Paterson-Brown S. Observation of behavioural markers of non-technical skills in the operating room and their relationship to intra-operative incidents. Surgeon. 2014 Jul 9. pii: S1479-666X(14)00075-4.
13. McCrory B, LaGrange CA, Hallbeck M. Quality and safety of minimally invasive surgery: past, present, and future. Biomed Eng Comput Biol. 2014;6:1–11.
14. Flin R, O'Connor P, Crichton M. Safety at the Sharp End: a guide to non-technical skills. Aldershot: Ashgate Publishing Limited; 2008.

15. Miskovic D, Wyles SM, Ni M, Darzi AW, Hanna GB. Systematic review on mentoring and simulation in laparoscopic colorectal surgery. Ann Surg. 2010;252(6):943–51.
16. Steinert Y, Mann K, Centeno A, et al. A systematic review of faculty development initiatives designed to improve teaching effectiveness in medical education: BEME Guide No. 8. Med Teach. 2006;28(6):497–526. doi:10.1080/01421590600902976.
17. Joint Advisory Group on GI Endoscopy. Secondary Joint Advisory Group on GI Endoscopy JAG Endoscopy Training System. http://www.jets.nhs.uk/.
18. Mackenzie H, Cuming T, Miskovic D, Wyles S, Langsford L, Valori R, Hanna GB, Coleman MG, Francis N. Design, delivery and validation of a training the trainer curriculum of in the English National Laparoscopic Colorectal Training Programme in England. Ann Surg. 2013;261(1):149–56.
19. Barnes RW. Surgical handcraft: teaching and learning surgical skills. Am J Surg. 1987;157:422–7.
20. Peyton J. The learning cycle. In: Peyton J, editor. Teaching and learning in medical practice. 1st ed. Guildford: Manticore Europe Limited; 1998. p. 1–12.
21. Ende J. Feedback in clinical medical education. JAMA. 1983;250:777–81.
22. Swinnen SP. Information feedback for motor skill learning: a review. In: Zelaznik N, editor. Advances in motor learning and control. Champaign: Human Kinetics press; 1996. p. 37–66.
23. Coderre S, Anderson J, Rostom A, Mclaughlin K. Training the endoscopy trainer: from general principles to specific concepts. Can J Gastroenterol. 2010;24(12):700–4.
24. Miskovic D, Wyles SM, Carter F, Coleman MG, Hanna GB. Development, validation and implementation of a monitoring tool for training in laparoscopic colorectal surgery in the English National Training Program. Surg Endosc. 2011;25(4):1136–42.
25. Mackenzie H, Miskovic D, Ni M, Parvaiz A, Acheson AG, Jenkins JT, Griffith J, Coleman MG, Hanna GB. Clinical and educational proficiency gain of supervised laparoscopic colorectal surgical trainees. Surg Endosc. 2013;27(8):2704–11.
26. Miskovic D, Ni M, Wyles SM, Kennedy RH, Francis NK, Parvaiz A, Cunningham C, Rockall TA, Gudgeon AM, Coleman MG, Hanna GB. National Training Programme in Laparoscopic Colorectal Surgery in England. Is competency assessment at the specialist level achievable? A study for the national training programme in laparoscopic colorectal surgery in England. Ann Surg. 2013;257(3):476–82.

Chapter 13
The Human Factor in Minimal Access Surgical Training: How Conscientious, Well-Trained Surgeons Make Mistakes

Rob Bethune and Nader Francis

Introduction

The former National Patient Safety Agency in the UK estimated that there are about three million admissions to NHS hospitals in England; of these about 300,000 will involve some sort of error that results in harm to a patient, and a further 30,000 patients will die as a result of those errors [1]. This is a higher number that equals the combined annual mortality from breast, prostate and colorectal cancer; a large problem [1]. The vast majority of these deaths are related to human factors and organisational systems so it logically follows that to reduce the number of errors and therefore harm, we need to focus on these areas and how we go about training surgeons to be more aware of their fallibility.

Surgery contributes to almost half of all adverse events and to 13 % of all hospital deaths. Some 40 % of these injuries are committed in the operating room (OR) [2]. Multiple estimates of adverse events in surgical patients have been undertaken and fairly consistently come up with a figure of 20 % [3, 4]. That means that 1 in 5 patients have an error in their care that results in harm of some kind and in 4 % the harm is so severe that they die. The conundrum is this; if surgeons are trained to a very high standard (which they are) so that they are equipped with the skills and knowledge to undertake the most difficult minimally access procedures (or any aspect of medicine for that matter), why do so many mistakes keep happening? The answer comes from further analysis of these errors. Retrospective reviews looking at

R. Bethune (✉)
Colorectal Surgery, Royal Devon and Exeter NHS Foundation Trust,
Barrack Road, Exeter, EX25DW, UK
e-mail: rob.bethune@nhs.net

N. Francis, MB ChB, PLAB, FRCS, PhD
Colorectal Surgery, Yeovil District Hospital NHS Foundation Trust,
Higher Kingston, Yeovil, Somerset BA21 4AT, UK
e-mail: Nader.francis@ydh.nhs.uk

N. Francis et al. (eds.), *Training in Minimal Access Surgery*,
DOI 10.1007/978-1-4471-6494-4_13

the underlying cause of these errors showed that only 6 % were related to a lack of knowledge and technical skill [4]. The surgical community can pat itself on the back and say that through the multiple training techniques that are detailed in the rest of this book they are very effective at making sure surgeons of the future are equipped with the technical skills they need. So what about the other 94 % of adverse events? The overwhelming majority (73 %) are related to the human factors that will be described in the rest of this book chapter, the remaining 20 % are related to organisational systems that made error extremely likely (i.e. having patients on non-specialist wards, saline and lignocaine in very similar bottles, etc.) [5, 6]. Although MAS carries significant benefits to the patient the operative environment imposes substantial physical and cognitive strain on the surgeon increasing the risk of error [6].

In this chapter the importance of human factors will be outlined as case presentations. The chapter also covers the various different components that make up human factors and finally how surgeons can be trained to be safer.

Story 1 – The Danger of Hierarchy

A consultant surgeon was performing a laparoscopic sigmoid colectomy to remove a malignant polyp in the distal sigmoid colon. The polyp had not been clearly tattooed so the surgeon performed an on-table colonoscopy to identify the site. He then used diathermy to mark the serosal surface. After mobilisation of the colon and division of the vessels he came on to dividing the bowel. He placed his stapler proximal to the mark he had made. The nurse softly said that she thought that the stapler was in the wrong place but the surgeon did not heed this comment and went on to divide the bowel. The nurse did not feel she could say anything more and that the surgeon must be right. On histological inspection it was clear that the line of transaction went across the polyp and the patient had to return to the OR for a further resection.

Human Factors

The term Human Factors (otherwise known as non-technical skills) relate to a variety of domains: communication, teamwork and leadership, decision making, situational awareness, stress and fatigue [7]. These traits are consistent across all human actions. Until recently most of the science relating to them came from industries outside health care, predominately aviation and the military.

Communication

Of all the domains of human factors communication is the most important and is the most significant factor in the majority of errors [8]. This is not a controversial statement; surgeons are well aware that communication is critical to good patient care

[9]. Despite this, very little emphasis is placed on inter-professional communication during undergraduate and post-graduate training. Healthcare tends to rest in a world of informal communication, where important messages are transmitted in haphazard ways that make mistakes almost certain. When OR performance is assessed at least 30 % of communication episodes result in failure visibly affecting system processes, including inefficiency, team tension, resource waste, delay and procedural error [8, 10, 11].

Structured, formalised communication results in better and safer care for patients [12]. Two recent examples of this are the WHO checklist (Box 13.1) and the SBAR tool (Box 13.2). Both of these systems originated in the aviation industry where they have been shown to reduce error and thereby the number of crashes and deaths. Formal communication like this is essential in healthcare but getting widespread adoption has been difficult. Most hospitals in the UK are using the WHO checklist in the peri-operative period but often these checks are not done properly and the full benefits are not realised [13].

Story 2 – Saved by a Flat Hierarchy

A consultant was supervising a trainee performing a laparoscopic appendicectomy. The patient's blood tests showed significantly raised inflammatory markers and on initial laparoscopy the pelvis contained significant amounts of turbid fluid. The appendix appeared mildly inflamed. The trainee performed the appedicectomy under close supervision. The consultant (who was distracted by thoughts of the complex laparotomy that would follow this case) told the trainee to wash out and close up. The trainee questioned this decision saying he was not happy that the appendix could explain the blood tests and the significant amount of turbid fluid. The consultant listened and heard what the trainee was suggesting and they then followed the small bowel along and found the real pathology, a perforated Meckel's diverticulum.

Operative briefings and debriefings are also now becoming common practice in the OR. These meetings allow the important points of the day to be discussed, thus improving efficiency and safety and, equally importantly, can influence the often steep hierarchy that exists in the OR [14, 15]. Although there was significant resistance to the initial implementation of pre-operative briefings, once they staff became familiar with them and the tangible benefits associated they have become a core component of most OR practice.

Team Working and Leadership

Nothing in healthcare is done by individuals alone; work is done in teams. It therefore follows that how these teams function is critical to the quality and safety of the care provided [16]. Surgeons work in multiple teams; in the OR, intensive care, surgical wards and the outpatients. Team members have to support each other, solve conflicts, exchange information and co-ordinate activities [7]. When successful teams are analysed, many factors are common, but the underlying factor without which teams cannot be successful is the interpersonal relationships that team members have. Without a harmonious group climate teams will never work to their optimal abilities. This is not to say that everyone has to be falsely nice to each other but if there is not mutual respect between all team members problems will occur.

As interpersonal relationships are so important major effort needs to be spent ensuring the strength of these relationships. Briefings, if done well, can contribute to this. Everyone must have a voice and feel that they contribute. At the start of effective briefings all staff must introduce themselves and by that very action of saying aloud their names they become more included and are more likely to speak up later if they have concerns.

Leadership is also crucial, not only by giving a clear direction to the tasks at hand but by ensuring that the authority gradient is kept to a minimum. There is no doubt that a team needs a leader on whom ultimate authority for decisions rest but the hierarchy around this needs to be kept at an absolute minimum. There are two problems with a steep authority gradient. Most obviously and dangerously if the people at the bottom of the hierarchy feel unable to speak up they will not bring potential safety problems to the group's attention. This has resulted in many incidents that have resulted in harm and death to patients. Stories 1 and 2 demonstrate the impact hierarchy can have. In the first story the nurse was well aware that the surgeon was dividing the bowel in the incorrect place but after softly mentioning it once, did not feel she could mention it again. In the second story the flatter hierarchy allowed the junior to speak up and prevent a potentially disastrous mistake from occurring. The OR team has many people in it and if they all feel that they can contribute to decision making and error prevention then patients will be safer.

Less well known is the impact that authority has on the leader. If someone exists at the top of a steep authority gradient their ability to understand and empathise with those beneath them diminishes, this has been shown in multiple behavioural science experients [17, 18]. So just by the act of promoting someone up the hierarchy the capacity to take appropriate decisions decreases.

Situational Awareness and Decision making

Situational awareness is the simple act of knowing what is going on around you and having an understanding of how that might change in the future. It is crucially important that all members of the team have the same understanding of what is going on; they share the same situational awareness. This is often not the case in the OR. This is another area where the pre-operative briefing can be helpful by ensuring that all members of the team are sharing the same understanding of the immediate world around them.

Story 3 – A Fatal Diagnostic Error

The on-call surgeon in a rural hospital in Eastern Africa was called in the early hours one morning. The message (which was hand delivered, there were no bleeps) stated that there was a 65 year old man in urinary retention but the night nurse could not catheterize the patient. The on-call surgeon went and briefly reviewed the patient at about 5-00 am. Urinary retention from benign prostatic hypertrophy (BPH) was a common diagnosis in the population the hospital served. The surgeon tried to catheterise the patient but could not get any urine back. The harder tipped catheters were kept in theatre which was locked and the on-call theatre team would have to be woken up. As the patient seemed reasonably comfortable the surgeon decided to give some analgesia and then sort the catheter out when the theatre opened at 8 am which was now only 2½ hours away.

When the patient was brought to theatre the surgeon immediately realised that the patient was now shocked and commenced resuscitation which was ultimately unsuccessful and the patient died. During the resuscitation it became clear that the diagnosis of benign prostatic hypertrophy was incorrect and in fact the patient has sigmoid volvulus and acute renal failure (hence no urine on catheterization).

Situation awareness forms the first part of the process of decision-making. Once information is taken in by the person or team then a series of potential options can be devised; one of these is selected and that becomes the plan. In story 3 the surgeon incorrectly assessed the situation; his situational awareness was wrong and so his decision-making process was fatally compromised. Why did the surgeon make the wrong assessment? There are several human factors that were at play but the most significant was the very common medical tendency of tunnel vision. The surgeon had been given the diagnosis, urinary retention secondarily to benign prostatic hypertrophy (BPH). It is a natural human tendency to try and fit the situation to our pre-conceived ideas. New information is accepted or rejected, based on how well it fits to the original thought; this is called conformational bias. In this case the surgeon noticed the facts that fitted his diagnosis; lower abdominal pain, no urine on catheterisation, and that the patient was the correct demographic for BPH. He disregarded, or paid less attention to, the facts that did not fit the diagnosis; lower blood pressure, tachycardia, tympanic abdomen and the fact that the catheter appeared to be going in smoothly. Earlier that day he had also managed a patient (correctly) with BPH; this tendency to diagnose recently seen conditions is called the availability heuristic.

We take decisions in two clearly distinct ways; Type 1 (fast) and Type 2 (slow). The classical medical diagnosis is made in the Type 2 or slow thinking mode. This is the deliberate and logical analysis of information and the construction of a series of differentials before performing examinations or tests to narrow the choices down to one favoured diagnosis. This systematic way is how all doctors were, and still are, taught at medical school. However, the reality is that doctors spend most of their time in Type 1, or fast thinking. This is the intuition or gut feelings that experienced doctors use when they see a patient and are presented with small amounts of information. They come to quick judgements that are very often correct and can allow them to make many decisions and review many patients in short periods of time. The problem with fast thinking is that it is much more susceptible to error due to the large number of cognitive biases that humans make. Clearly the surgeon in the clinical case of story 3 was thinking in the Type 1 mode. Fast thinking is essentially to delivering timely care and should continue, but the clinician needs to be aware of the significant impact of cognitive bias.

Stress, Fatigue and Distraction

The other significant factor underlying the fatal error in story 3 is fatigue. The surgeon was woken from sleep at 5 a.m., he was doing a 1:2 on-call rota covering obstetrics and general surgery for a population of two million people and was chronically exhausted. The simple fact is that when surgeons are tired they are more likely to make mistakes. There is nothing that can be done to change this except recognising it, communicating the problem to other members of the team so that they are aware, and to try and avoid difficult decisions when they are tired. After 17 h without sleep (a night on-call) decision-making and procedural ability equates with being just over the legal alcohol limit for driving in the UK. This situation is clearly of relevance to advanced laparoscopic surgery, *e.g.* laparoscopic rectal surgery in obese males who have had neo-adjuvant chemo-radiotherapy. By the time the surgeon has completed the first part of the operation (dissection of the vascular pedicle and mobilisation of the splenic flexure) his or her level of concentration and attention will inevitably be reduced. The surgeon is then faced with the most challenging part of the operation, to remove the rectal cancer safely from the narrow and deep pelvis and without compromising the oncological quality of the specimen or the pelvic nerves. The surgeon needs to rest at this point to reduce the chance of an error. This can either be done by taking time out (leaving the sterile field and having a quick drink), or by handing over to another equally competent surgeon. This concept of dual operating is likely to become more frequent as more complex and long operations are undertaken with MAS.

Story 4 – The Danger of Distraction

A newly appointed consultant surgeon was performing a laparoscopic oesphagectomy and was suturing the oesphago-gastric anastomosis. This is a very technically demanding part of the operation. When the back wall of the anastomosis was being sutured, a senior consultant put his head round the door (behind the operating surgeon) and checked that things were going all-right. The two surgeons had a brief chat and then the operating surgeon continued to suture. During the conversation the suture had been dropped and when the next stitch was placed it had been locked (the threads crossed over preventing it being pulled tight). The surgeon had to then unpick the thread which proved difficult and then carry on with the anastomosis. Three days later this anastomosis leaked from exactly that spot and the patient had to return to the OR and have an oesophagostomy.

Stress and distraction also degrade our cognitive abilities. This is significant for everyone, but can have specific problems related to surgical training. If a surgical trainee has to cover both the management of ward patients and then go to the OR to operate his or her ability to learn will be reduced. After a busy ward round with multiple problems and associated tasks, it is impossible for the trainee to completely put these out of his or her mind and so will be distracted by them; this is called dual system interference and is a significant problem across healthcare. The other common example in the OR is noise distraction. In story 4 the operating surgeon was distracted at the crucial part of the operation. Although the subsequent leak could not be definitely put down to the interruption it is likely that it contributed to it. Compared to the other domains of human factors, reducing distraction in the OR should be a relatively easy situation to improve. For example, no OR staff should have their mobile phones whilst surgery is being performed and no-one should be allowed to enter the OR during crucial parts of the operation.

Dual Task Interference and Training

All humans have a variable, but limited, capacity to perform cognitive and manual tasks. Whilst performing a manual task if a significant cognitive burden is placed on the operator then that manual performance will degrade. Think of trying to juggle whilst counting backwards, humans cannot do both well. The more familiar the task and the more practiced the individual, the greater the ability to maintain performance in the presence of additional sensory stimuli. Therefore external interference will affect novices and trainees more significantly than experts; however experts can be, and still are affected by distraction. Examples of interference include auditory distraction, *e.g.* music, conversation, radio pagers and telephones and visual distraction by movement of people or objects in the field of vision. The impact of the distraction will depend on the amount of cognition needed to deal with it. Quiet music will have considerably less impact than a direct question to the operator.

Trainers should effectively control the OR environment to reduce interference and distraction whilst the trainee is operating.

How Can We Train Surgeons to Be Safer?

Human factors are intrinsic weaknesses and therefore they are as impossible to eradicate as error is itself. The question is how can surgeons be trained to make fewer errors and how can systems be designed that make errors harder to make?

Lessons from the Aviation Industry

Story 5 – The World's Worst Airline Crash
In Tenerife in 1977 two Boeing 747 s were taxing on the runway on a foggy day. The captain of the KLM flight (who was the most experienced pilot in the fleet) thought he heard from the air traffic controllers say that he was clear for take-off; in fact they had only asked if they were ready for take-off. The Pam Am flight was still on the main runway and told the air traffic controllers that they were not clear. The flight engineer on the KLM flight asked the captain 'are they not clear then', the captain emphatically over ruled this and carried on with the take-off. The planes collided on the runway and 583 people died.

During the 1970s the aviation industry responded to a series of high profile crashes, including the one described, caused by human error rather than equipment failure [15]. The industry implemented a programme called Crew Resource Management (CRM) training. This was a comprehensive programme in which all airline crews, pilots and cabin crew were trained in human factors. Through a series of lectures, workshops and simulator training all staff were exposed and assessed on their ability to communicate and work in teams. This then became a mandatory requirement and airline staff are now annually trained and assessed. Staff, particularly senior pilots, who were not prepared to accept the new flat hierarchies and culture were dismissed, although in practice this rarely happened. As a result of this industry-wide, decade long effort the number of crashes and deaths relating to human error decreased significantly. In addition to individual and team training the aviation industry implemented a series of system changes that made errors harder to make. Much of this was related to conducting formal briefings, debriefings and checklists. Story 5 shows how steep the hierarchy was in the aviation industry in the 1970s; the flight engineer questioned the captain about the radio message but the captain paid no heed to this and the engineer did not feel he could persist in questioning his senior, note the similarities to Story 1. As a result of the subsequent inquest the language that pilots and air traffic controllers could use became much more standardised reducing the chance of similar confusion. The word 'take-off' was banned for all uses except for when a plane was cleared for take-off. Had this been in place it is likely that the Tenerife crash would not have happened. Currently this kind of standardised language does not exist uniformly in healthcare exposing patients to the possibility of harm from communication error. Box 13.2 describes the SBAR format for handover which is an example that is beginning to be used in healthcare to standardise communication.

Team Training in Healthcare

In an effort to replicate the huge improvements in the aviation industry a variety of team training systems have developed following the CRM example. These take a variety of forms, including formal teaching on human factors and simulation training. Different training programs have been developed as well as methods to evaluate human factors [19, 20]. As yet none of these programmes have become sufficiently widespread in healthcare or proved as effective as the CRM airline training.

The most widely implemented programme is the Team STEPPS programme from the United States. This programme was developed jointly by the American Department of Defence and the Agency for Healthcare Research and Quality. A series of different levels of human factor training is provided within a hospital. A detailed 2-day course is run for a small cadre of leaders, who will go on to deliver the other phases of training. All clinical staff then receive 4–6 h of workshop based training and then all non-clinical support staff receive 2 h of training. Team STEPPS has been evaluated in a variety of studies and consistently shows an improvement in team work behaviours [21, 22], but as yet no studies have been done to show that this has resulted in safer and more effective care for patients.

In the Severn Deanery (Bristol, UK) all surgical trainees receive a full day of training on human factors using simulation-based training. Each domain is introduced to the group and then a simulation session is run on a mock ward with most of the trainees watching through a one way glass screen and the others actively participating in the simulation. Situations are created that bring out the various domains of human factors, for example using distraction to induce an error. The use of simulation increases the fidelity of the training.

Training Briefings

The impact of pre-operative briefings is clear for patients and the OR team. With a simple addition to this the briefing can be a very useful tool to help trainees learn as well. At the University Hospital Bristol NHS Foundation Trust a trial of training briefings was conducted [23]. During the briefing the training surgeon made it clear to the trainee or trainees which part of the operation they would be doing. For example in reference to an laparoscopic anterior resection they might have said ‘the junior trainee will achieve access into the abdomen, then the more senior trainee will perform the left sided mobilisation of the colon including the splenic flexure and then the consultant surgeon will perform the rectal dissection'. This kind of training briefing can encourage a dialogue between trainee and trainer, helping to ensure that specific training needs can be addressed and progress measured in conjunction with the surgical curriculum. Moreover, it provides trainees with a defined, tangible role in the OR environment regardless of the complexity of the operation, eliminating the normal worries about being excluded from 'doing' any of the operation. Training briefings also provide the OR team with a clear plan. By and large, trainees take longer to complete any aspect of a procedure compared with their consultant colleagues, which can cause difficulties for the staff responsible for managing the list and its resources. By dividing the operation into smaller components, this can largely be mitigated. Additionally, the training briefing includes a strategy delineating the point at which the trainer will take over if required. This is not only helpful for the OR staff but also for the trainees, because rather than being perceived as constituting failure, it becomes an expected and predictable event [23].

The Debrief: The Key to Learning and Improving

Debriefing at the end of a OR list is both one of the most important communication episodes in the OR day and simultaneously one of the least done. In the author's anecdotal experience it is unusual for a debriefing to take place after a OR list. Time pressures and a lack of perceived importance often combine to prevent this happening. This is a great lost opportunity as the debrief is the moment when a team can learn and improve. At the debrief the team can discuss their performance during the day. This is often best lead by a senior member of the team describing some aspect of the day's performance that could have been improved and discussing potential ways in which this could occur (i.e. the surgeon changing the order of the list on the day for a reason that could have been predicted). This can then encourage others to speak about their own areas for improvement. This meeting needs to be largely positive and works best when people talk about their own errors. If it turns into a meeting where one person criticises or blames the others, then the debrief can have a negative impact on the interpersonal relationships that underpin any successful team.

The Way Forward

The world is already changing. The fact that a manual on surgical training in minimal access surgery contains a chapter on human factors shows how far this field has moved. Five years ago human factors were very rarely talked about in medicine and surgery and certainly few healthcare-related training programs existed. This progress needs to be built on. All surgeons need to be exposed to human factors training, preferably in the teams that they work in. By doing this a huge number of deaths and adverse events that are happening every day will be reduced and the care provided to patients will become safer and more efficient.

Box 13.1: The WHO Safer Surgery Checklist

Atul Gawande and colleagues trialled what has now become the WHO safer surgery checklist. Their intervention included team training and the use of the pre-operative briefings. The study was carried out in four developing world and four developed world hospitals. Seven thousand operations were observed, half before the introduction and half after. The mortality was reduced by 46 % and the morbidity by 36 % when the checklist was used. Both results were statistically significant. The study was published as a paper in the New England Journal of Medicine in 2009.

The checklist has been made mandatory across the NHS in the UK, but in most cases when the checklist was implemented it was not accompanied by the team training that was provided in the research study and as such the significant benefits for patients that were seem in the trial may not occur with the checklist alone.

Box 13.2: The SBAR Communication Tool

The SBAR (Situation, Background, Assessment and Recommendation) Tool was developed to formalise communications and help both the sender and the receiver to transmit meaning accurately. It consists of four parts:-

S – Situation

A brief outline of the current state of the patient ('Mr Y is tachycardic and sweaty')

B – Background

What has happened running up to this moment? ('Mr Y was previously fit and well and had a right hemi-colectomy for cancer this morning')

A – Assessment

The state of play now. ('His HR is 130, his BP is 110/80. I think he is in shock and has already received 2 l of fluid')

R – Recommendation

What the sender wants the receiver to do ('Can you come to ward 7A immediately as I think he is bleeding and needs to go back to theatre').

References

1. Mortality Statistics, Office of National Statistics. 2008.
2. Tang B, Hanna GB, Joice P, Cuschieri A. Identification and categorization of technical errors by Observational Clinical Human Reliability Assessment (OCHRA) during laparoscopic cholecystectomy. Arch Surg. 2004;139(11):1215–20.

3. Kable AK, Gibberd RW, Spigelman AD. Adverse events in surgical patients in Australia. Int J Qual Health Care. 2002;14(4):269–76.
4. van Wagtendonk I, Smits M, Merten H, Heetveld MJ, Wagner C. Nature, causes and consequences of unintended events in surgical units. Br J Surg. 2010;97(11):1730–40.
5. Siu J, Maran N, Paterson-Brown S. Observation of behavioural markers of non-technical skills in the operating room and their relationship to intra-operative incidents. Surgeon. 2014. [Epub ahead of print].
6. McCrory B, LaGrange CA, Hallbeck M. Quality and safety of minimally invasive surgery: past, present, and future. Biomed Eng Comput Biol. 2014;6:1–11.
7. Flin R, O'Connor P, Crichton M. Safety at the Sharp End: a guide to non-technical skills. Burlington: Ashgate Publishing Limited, Surrey GU97PT, England; 2008.
8. Gawande AA, Zinner MJ, Studdert DM, Brennan TA. Analysis of errors reported by surgeons at three teaching hospitals. Surgery. 2003;133(6):614–21.
9. Baldwin PJ, Paisley AM, Brown SP. Consultant surgeons' opinion of the skills required of basic surgical trainees. Br J Surg. 1999;86(8):1078–82.
10. Christian CK, Gustafson ML, Roth EM, Sheridan TB, Gandhi TK, Dwyer K, et al. A prospective study of patient safety in the operating room. Surgery. 2006;139(2):159–73.
11. Lingard L, Espin S, Whyte S, Regehr G, Baker GR, Reznick R, et al. Communication failures in the operating room: an observational classification of recurrent types and effects. Qual Saf Health Care. 2004;13(5):330–4.
12. Haynes AB, Weiser TG, Berry WR, Lipsitz SR, Breizat AH, Dellinger EP, et al. A surgical safety checklist to reduce morbidity and mortality in a global population. N Engl J Med. 2009;360(5):491–9.
13. Braaf S, Manias E, Riley R. The 'time-out' procedure: an institutional ethnography of how it is conducted in actual clinical practice. BMJ Qual Saf. 2013;22(8):647–55.
14. Ali M, Osborne A, Bethune R, Pullyblank A. Preoperative surgical briefings do not delay operating room start times and are popular with surgical team members. J Patient Saf. 2011;7(3):139–43.
15. Bethune R, Sasirekha G, Sahu A, Cawthorn S, Pullyblank A. Use of briefings and debriefings as a tool in improving team work, efficiency, and communication in the operating theatre. Postgrad Med J. 2011;87(1027):331–4.
16. Cuschieri A. Nature of human error: implications for surgical practice. Ann Surg. 2006;244(5):642–8.
17. Galinsky AD, Magee JC, Inesi ME, Gruenfeld DH. Power and perspectives not taken. Psychol Sci. 2006;17(12):1068–74.
18. Kraus M, Piff P, Keltner D. Social class as culture: the convergence of resources and rank in the social realm. Curr Direct Psychol Sci. 2011;20:246–50.
19. McCulloch P, Mishra A, Handa A, Dale T, Hirst G, Catchpole K. The effects of aviation-style non-technical skills training on technical performance and outcome in the operating theatre. Qual Saf Health Care. 2009;18(2):109–15.
20. Crossley J, Marriott J, Purdie H, Beard JD. Prospective observational study to evaluate NOTSS (Non-Technical Skills for Surgeons) for assessing trainees' non-technical performance in the operating theatre. Br J Surg. 2011;98(7):1010–20.
21. Meier AH, Boehler ML, McDowell CM, Schwind C, Markwell S, Roberts NK, et al. A surgical simulation curriculum for senior medical students based on TeamSTEPPS. Arch Surg. 2012;147(8):761–6.
22. Lisbon D, Allin D, Cleek C, Roop L, Brimacombe M, Downes C, et al. Improved knowledge, attitudes, and behaviors after implementation of TeamSTEPPS Training in an Academic Emergency Department: a pilot report. Am J Med Qual. 2014. [Epub ahead of print].
23. Bethune R, Blencowe NS. The trainee's voice: recognising the importance of preoperative briefings for surgical trainees. J Perioper Pract. 2014;24(3):56–8.

Index

N. Francis et al. (eds.), *Training in Minimal Access Surgery*,
DOI 10.1007/978-1-4471-6494-4

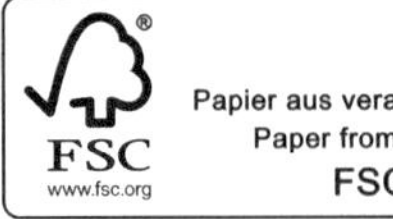

If you have any concerns about our products, you can contact us on
ProductSafety@springernature.com

In case Publisher is established outside the EU, the EU authorized representative is:
Springer Nature Customer Service Center GmbH
Europaplatz 3, 69115 Heidelberg, Germany

Printed by Libri Plureos GmbH
in Hamburg, Germany